Praise for Peggy Brill's
The Core Program

"Nothing is more important to strength, health, and vitality than strong core muscles. I know this from both personal and professional experience. Peggy Brill's exercise program is effective for every woman, no matter what her current fitness level. And because it takes only 15 minutes per day, everyone can benefit."

—Christiane Northrup, M.D.,
author of *Women's Bodies, Women's Wisdom*

"I never thought I'd be free from back pain due to arthritis and hard living for my first forty years. Now forty-nine, I started the Core Program three and a half weeks ago and have just had four days in a row with absolutely NO PAIN! I'm ecstatic. I'm starting to believe my second forty years will be enjoyable after all!" —Kathy Okay

"I am fifteen and in high school. I have gradually worked my way up to the Ultimate Core and have seen myself get more flexible and toned. I have recommended this program to my mom (age fifty), sister (age twelve), grandma (age eighty-one), and several of my friends and they have gotten excellent results too!"

—A reader from Glenview, Illinois, on Amazon

"I'm not very flexible and am constantly lifting my sixteen-month-old daughter. Needless to say, my back is continually aching. Even though I've only been doing this program for a week, already the soreness is diminished to the point where it is almost gone. I really thought I would have to deal with back pain for the rest of my life. What a relief, in more ways than one, to know I can do something about it. As an added bonus, my stomach is getting flatter—something that hasn't happened since before I was pregnant!"

—A reader from Pittsburgh, on Amazon

"Working with Peggy Brill is a dream! Her ideas are terrific . . . she makes you feel confident about improvement."

—Mike Krzyzewski (aka Coach K),
Duke University Men's Basketball

"*The Core Program* is for everyone who wants to enjoy optimum health over the course of a lifetime."

—Charles B. Goodwin, M.D.,
The Hospital for Special Surgery (New York, NY)

"I only wish I had met Peggy while in my twenties. Peggy is new science—and her program is the best and safest way to turn back the clock and start feeling fabulous."

—Lauren Hutton, model

Also by Peggy W. Brill, P.T.

THE CORE PROGRAM
15 Minutes a Day
That Can Change Your Life

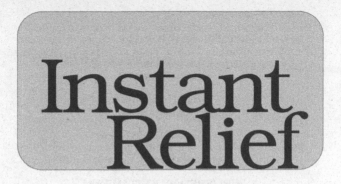

Instant Relief

Tell me where it **hurts**
and I'll tell you what to do

Peggy W. Brill, P.T.

with Susan Suffes

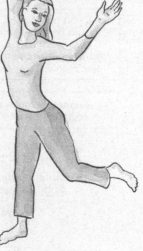

BANTAM BOOKS
New York Toronto London Sydney Auckland

The exercises and suggestions in this book are guidelines for the healthy individual. If you have specific medical problems or are unsure whether you should perform certain exercises, please consult your physician or physical therapist.

INSTANT RELIEF
A Bantam Book

PUBLISHING HISTORY
Bantam trade paperback edition published June 2003
Bantam mass market edition/January 2008

PUBLISHED BY BANTAM DELL
A Division of Random House, Inc.
New York, New York

Bantam Books and the rooster colophon are registered trademarks of Random House, Inc.

ISBN 978-0-553-58547-6

Printed in the United States of America
Published simultaneously in Canada

www.bantamdell.com

For my greatest love and joy,

Madison and Maggie

Contents

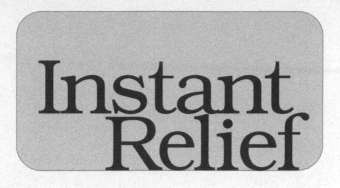

Instant Relief

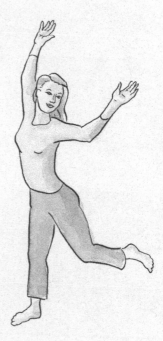

Introduction

Everyone knows that it is impossible to control all the stress that is an inevitable part of our daily lives. But stress-induced *pain* is another matter. The good news is that we *can* do something to control those sudden onsets of pain and discomfort, *whenever* and *wherever* they occur. You can get *Instant Relief* with the Brill exercises. A few simple movements—and relief is yours.

The fact that emotional stress can cause physical pain was never more evident to me than after the events of September 11, 2001. As a physical therapist practicing in Manhattan, I found that within forty-eight hours I was dealing with an epidemic of physical problems.

A Head-Spine Analogy

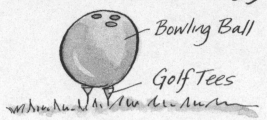

Bowling Ball

Golf Tees

Patients were phoning or just showing up with complaints about sudden unrelenting pain in all parts of their bodies. Necks were stiff. Backs were aching. Shoulders were tense. Knees and hips were sore. Over and over again I heard about pain that seemed to strike out of nowhere, almost all of it a manifestation of the emotional upheaval an entire nation was experiencing.

Pain occurs because part of the body's first-wave response to emotional stress is to tense the muscles. Certain muscles are particularly predisposed to this tightening, especially those in the upper neck, the shoulders, the jaw, and the muscles along the spine. In the lower back the connective tissue becomes tense and tight, too. When muscles and connective tissue tighten, nerves may become entrapped and blood flow becomes constricted, cutting off the oxygen and nutrients the muscles need. A neck ache or a backache is sure to follow.

The diaphragm, a key respiratory muscle

located at the bottom of the rib cage, also responds to stress by tightening. Think about a time when you were under stress. How did you breathe? Unless you consciously made the decision to take the deep diaphragmatic breaths your body needed, you probably took rapid, shallow breaths, inhaling too little oxygen and exhaling incompletely so that your lungs did not make room for even the limited amount of oxygen you were inhaling. You may have noticed that your hands and feet were cold—a sure sign that not enough blood was circulating to your extremities. This is because shallow breathing constricts blood vessels, further contributing to the cutting off of the blood supply that is caused by the tightening of the other muscles in the body.

Headaches, backaches, neck pain, tingling and numbness in the hands—these are only some of the possible results of muscle tension and shallow breathing. Conversely, all of them can be relieved by proper breathing, and by balancing muscles through the stretching and strengthening exercises I'll be giving you in this book.

Stress is—and always has been—everywhere. It's in our offices, in our homes, in our relationships—and now more than ever, it's in the scary new world outside our front door. But stress is an inevitable part of the human condition, even in the best of times. So let's accept that fact, even as we focus on learning

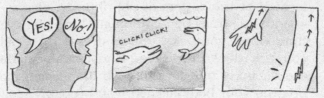

Human Speak   Dolphin Speak   Body Speak

how to reject pain, its consequence. We *can* get rid of pain.

But first we should listen to it. Pain is the body's alarm system to warn us that something is being injured. Learning how to respond to the warning signs of pain is what the one hundred Brill exercises are all about. Using them in my physical therapy practice, I've treated thousands of patients successfully.

So just show me where it hurts, and I'll tell you what to do. A simple ten-second exercise could be all you need to put an end to your pain. That's what Instant Relief is all about.

Emotional or Physical: Stress Hurts

Sometimes stress-induced pain comes on suddenly, as when there is a crisis at work or a medical emergency affecting someone you love. At other times pain is the result of more chronic, ongoing situations, such as a job you really hate or a conflict between you and a spouse or a child. And sometimes pain has an immediate physical cause. A spur-of-the-moment decision on the first day of spring to

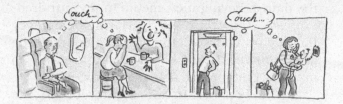

go out and play eighteen holes of golf after a sedentary winter is just as likely to result in pain as fear of flying, anxiety about losing money in the stock market, or tension in one of your relationships. *The body does not distinguish between emotional and physical triggers.*

Every day there are endless potential causes for the onset of sudden pain. There's the unexpected twinge in your shoulder as you lift the baby's stroller onto the bus. A hip pain grips you when you're playing a pickup game of basketball. The lightning-bolt headache strikes just as you're about to give the make-or-break presentation at the business meeting you've spent three months preparing for.

You know only too well what it's like to feel trapped, whether in a doctor's waiting room, at a PTA meeting, in a cramped seat on a long flight, on a kitchen stool while visiting an argumentative relative, or stuck in your car in a traffic jam. The result is an unbearably awful combination of physical discomfort, hard-to-control anger, and ever-increasing anxiety. But now, whenever you end up in one of these dreaded situations, you can use one or more of the pain-relieving movements in my hundred-exercise repertoire to perform emergency therapy on yourself. You can give yourself the gift of *Instant Relief* wherever you are and no matter what you are doing.

Maybe you are in an elevator or on the street, in a theater or on a train or bus, when pain strikes. You press your fingers to your temples in an attempt to ease your suddenly throbbing head. Or you stop dead in the middle of a game of tennis to rub an aching knee. After hours of sitting at your desk you get up and immediately begin to self-massage your back. But these strategies rarely work.

Wouldn't you prefer to use actions that are proven to provide the relief you seek? Based on results with thousands of patients, the emergency therapy in *Instant Relief* will help you minimize stress-induced pain at any hour of the night or day and in whatever situation you find yourself. Soon you'll know how to stop the needless suffering!

Emergency Therapy When and Where You Need It

I know that stress-induced pain is not restricted to just a few areas of the body. That's why I'm going to give you a hundred easy-to-do movements that work on all the parts vulnerable to pain, including:

- Head
- Neck

- Shoulders
- Elbows
- Hands
- Mid-back
- Lower back
- Hips
- Knees
- Calves
- Feet

With my Brill exercises you will be able to make the correction you need the moment you need it. And all of these exercises are not only effective but fast. You'll either repeat one small movement ten times, or you'll do the movement once and hold it for ten seconds. That's all there is to it. A small investment—a huge return!

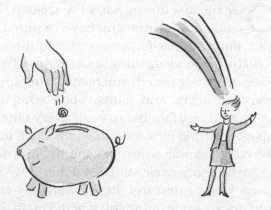

Small Investment (vs.) *Huge Gain*

When stress pain strikes, you may be talking on a phone, standing at a reception, sitting at your child's recital, or in one of dozens of other situations that require you to remain where you are. Most of the simple movements I'm going to give you will enable you to do just that.

- If you are standing, I'll show you a variety of easy movements to alleviate your pain right where you are.
- If you are sitting, I'll put dozens of pain-killing antidotes at your disposal without asking you to get out of your chair.
- If you are lying in your bed, you'll be able to obtain relief without getting up.

I Know the Brill Exercises Work

Over the last fifteen years I've treated thousands of patients who have required regular, ongoing care for a variety of injuries and structural abnormalities. But many of them have also requested emergency therapy for everyday aches and pains. Their complaints will sound very familiar to you. "Every time I get up after sitting for a long time, my back hurts" is a common one; so are "Whenever I'm stuck in a meeting, my neck starts to ache," "My knee hurts when I descend steps," and "My calves and toes cramp at night when I'm in bed." Working with these patients, I've developed an extensive repertoire of easy techniques that often help them to relieve discomfort within seconds. The Brill exercises work for them, and they'll work for you, too.

Many of these exercises have also been effective for patients suffering from chronic pain when stress has worsened their condition. People with cancer, coronary artery disease, osteoarthritis, migraines, and other conditions have found quick relief with these Brill exercises, which not only alleviate their discomfort but also reassure them that the pain they are feeling is not caused by their underlying disease. These simple interventions go a long way toward helping them feel a lot better.

I also prescribe Brill exercises to post-op patients who are facing months of physical therapy. For instance, I see a number of people who have had back surgery, especially a *microdiskectomy*, which involves removing a piece of displaced disk from the back. When these patients start to experience lower-back pain, they use the Brill exercises that specifically target their pain, whether they are sitting, standing, or lying down.

Here's one example. Bill, a forty-two-year-old accountant, came to me six months after a microdiskectomy. "I thought the operation would relieve my pain," he told me, "but I'm still feeling that annoying localized lower-back discomfort I felt prior to my surgery. I've run the gamut of anti-inflammatories, and their side effects are really bothering me. What can I do now?"

I told him to do the Pelvic Rock (Exercise 49) once an hour while sitting at his desk. And although he gave me a somewhat skeptical look, he followed my advice. One week later he told me, "I can't believe it. I did just what you told me to do, and it worked each time. As days went by, I didn't need to do the exercise as often. Now I know that whenever I feel a twinge, I can take care of it myself by performing certain exercises."

My quick fixes, which are based on a sound understanding of anatomy and physiology, help people like Bill every day—and they can help you, too.

Stop Pain Before It Becomes Chronic

Your body is affected constantly by a number of mechanical stresses—frequently repeated movements, and long-held, out-of-balance postures—that also create discomfort.

For the millions of you who are what I call "computer jocks," mechanical stresses are a real problem. You sit at a desk most of the day, but nature built you to be mobile. Staying in one position for long periods of time doesn't allow optimal blood circulation to all areas of the body. You're also likely to use the same muscles over and over—think about all the mouse-clicking and phone-hugging you do—but nature intended you to use your muscles symmetrically, with one set of muscles balancing another.

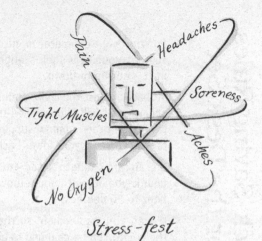

Stress-fest

Sitting at a computer for hours on end can distort the proper alignment of the shoulders, the neck, the back, the wrists and hands, and even the knees and hips. Over time your body will pay a toll for these static, out-of-alignment positions. Some muscles will tend to shorten and tighten, while others will lengthen and weaken. When this happens, pain kicks in, which is the body's built-in alarm system—a surefire indicator of dysfunction. (See my first book, *The Core Program,* for detailed advice and illustrations for how to set up your desk, chair, phone, reading material, and computer monitor and keyboard to avoid these problems.)

Slouching causes pain, too, and for similar reasons: some muscles become short and tight, while the opposite muscles become long

1. Position your computer monitor so that your eyes look straight at it—not up or down.

2. Sit back against the chair, preferably with a small pillow, rolled-up towel, or other lumbar support for the curve in your lower back.

3. Sit an arms-length away from your keyboard, with your elbows bent to 90 degrees.

4. Use an adjustable chair, so that the height can be changed to allow for your knees to be at a 90-degree angle to your hips, when your feet are flat on the floor.

5. And, in the best of all possible worlds, you will use a telephone headset, so that you don't have to bend your neck to a receiver.

and weak from overstretching. When you slouch for an extended period of time, for example while hunching over a project you're working on at your desk, your breathing may also be affected, because your diaphragm is compressed, making it difficult to breathe deeply. Not only are you taxing certain muscles, you're cutting off the supply of oxygen you need to nourish every cell in your body, from your brain to your toes.

Another potential problem occurs if most of your desk equipment is set up on one side, because then you'll end up having to favor one side of your body. That means the muscles on the other side are going to weaken from lack of use. And guess what? Your joints are going to start to hurt because of the mechanical imbalances of muscles pulling on them asymmetrically.

For all the reasons described above, the Brill exercises have been designed to ensure that your muscles are balanced and your body is in alignment, so that your joints will spin, glide, and roll through their optimal range of motion. Another benefit of the Brill exercises is that if the joints move as they should, the cartilage, which covers and cushions the joint surfaces and also produces synovial fluid for friction-free motion along the joint surfaces, won't wear down. This, in turn, will help to prevent osteoarthritis.

Don't Wait Until Pain Strikes

I'm going to give you simple techniques to offset the strains that accumulate in your body every day because of poor posture during work, play, and even sleep. The Brill exercises will stretch muscles that have gotten tight, move your body in ways that will restore muscle balance, and thereby help to put a stop to the degenerative changes that come from misuse and aging. You'll feel better fast.

But you don't have to wait until pain strikes to do the Brill exercises; you can employ them as a first line of defense against injury. *The stronger and better balanced the muscles of your body are to begin with, the less likely you will feel stress-induced pain.* So think of these exercises not just as a curative, but as a preventative as well.

These small interventions really work. I've had seventy-year-old patients come to me complaining of pains they've experienced for ten or even twenty years. Now their pains are gone. They've learned that they can control the stresses and strains on their bodies, counteract them, and live pain-free. This is my dream: to change how we age so that we don't have to suffer with the pain that is too often considered a normal part of aging.

Listen to Your Body

Instead of trying to ignore pain, I'm going to suggest that you pay more attention to it, because then you'll be able to do something to relieve it. By learning to listen to your body, you'll discover that you can head off little annoyances before they become big problems. I've organized the exercises in this book by body part. So if your neck begins to bother you, for example, you can go directly to the *Instant Relief* neck exercises.

Although the little movements in these Brill exercises seem so simple that it's hard to believe they could have an effect, if you repeat them several times throughout the day you'll be stretching, strengthening, and rebalancing your muscles, and you'll be amazed at how quickly they eliminate pain. Doesn't it make sense to take control of your discomfort instead of letting it increase to the point where it lands you in bed or on anti-inflammatories or painkillers?

Focusing on the cause of pain is the most direct way of alleviating discomfort. When my older daughter was four years old and had tummyaches, I showed her that rubbing her belly counterclockwise, from the right side to the top, to the left side and then to the bottom, would help. And while she didn't know that the motion followed the path of the ascending, transverse, and descending portions of the colon, thereby helping to move food particles through the digestive tract, she knew it worked. Now whenever her tummy hurts, she knows what to do.

If a four-year-old can isolate her pain and learn to rid herself of it in seconds, so can you. These simple ten-second movements will also help you to stay active. I know that many people limit their physical activities once they feel pain, but that only adds to their problem. Once you stop exercising, the muscles in your body become even more imbalanced. Using *Instant Relief*, you'll be able to eliminate your pain quickly and get back to walking, running, playing sports, and all the other things that are part of a healthy lifestyle. But even if you never exercise, don't worry. The movements described in this book are easy to do, and they will work for you, too.

Here are two variations of an exercise that I find amazingly effective for most neck and arm pain. I prescribe it routinely for many patients, especially those who spend hours on the phone and/or working at computers. Not only does the exercise relieve their pain, it makes them smile, too.

Please note that both Brill Chicken movements are an exception to the *Instant Relief* exercises, which generally consist of small, barely noticeable movements that will not draw attention to what you're doing. I can understand not wanting to perform a Brill Chicken at a four-star restaurant while you are entertaining your number-one client, or on the dais at your parents' fortieth wedding anniversary party. On the other hand, you can

About That Brill Dead Chicken

Don't laugh.. it works!

You can do these movements sitting or standing. Sure they look funny—but they feel *so* good. Here's what you do:

- Tuck in your chin and pull your head back, elongating the back of your neck.
- Push out your chest and lift it, pinching your shoulder blades together.
- Bend your arms and pull your hands back toward your shoulders, keeping your elbows close to your torso and your palms facing outward. Hold for a count of ten, and release.

1. Brill Chicken

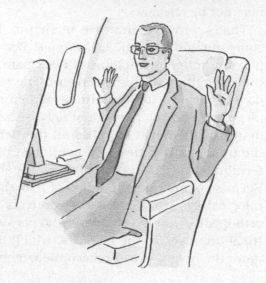

always excuse yourself, go to the restroom, and do it. Or get *everyone* to do it, and share the instant relief—and some laughter.

The Science Behind the Solution

The Brill exercises work because they are based on a deep understanding of the biomechanical and biochemical reactions that help the human body to function. You may wonder how stretching your thighs will help your aching knees or what pulling your shoulder blades together has to do with a sore neck. Years as a physical therapist have shown me how the integrated systems of the body interact and how they affect one another. I always look for the underlying dysfunction that is causing the pain, even though the connection may not be obvious.

That's why patients are often puzzled by some of my diagnostic techniques. For example, if a patient complains of neck pain, I test the strength of his or her fingers. The reason I do this pertains to the anatomy of the brachial plexus, which is a network of nerves that originates in the neck, supplies all the nerves to the upper extremities, and continues to three terminal branches that end in the hands. Because of my understanding of how the neurological system of the body connects to the orthopedic system—the nerves generate electrical impulses to the muscles, which in turn move the bones—I can determine which nerve in the neck is affected by seeing which finger is not functioning properly.

The point is that I know where your pain is coming from—and I will give you the simplest, most effective movements to treat it at the source, which is the best way to knock it out. So take this book with you wherever you go. That way you'll always have the Brill exercises on hand; ready with the help you need, when you need it. Instead of masking a symptom with an over-the-counter pain medication, you can reach for *Instant Relief*.

The Relief You Need, When You Need It

It doesn't matter whether you're a patient of mine coming in for three sessions of physical therapy a week, a daily follower of the exercise regimen I described in *The Core Program*, or someone who never exercises at all. During the course of any given day or week you are likely to feel some kind of stress-induced pain. Your life is full of challenges—and they are not going to disappear. Olympic athletes, computer jocks, weekend golfers, high-pressured executives, and stay-at-home parents alike will find in this book an easy way to counteract pain whenever and wherever it strikes.

I believe that good health is a gift. It's time to celebrate the divine workings of your body and tend to its needs daily with *Instant Relief*.

Muscle Soreness

It is completely typical to feel a bit of discomfort when you first do some of the Brill exercises, because the movements stretch abnormally tight tissues to their normal length. Over time the discomfort should diminish, however, because the more you stretch those tense muscles, the less tight they'll be. If, however, you find that the discomfort is not lessening, perform the exercise with less intensity in a range that is tolerable for you.

If a sore muscle persists, you can apply a covered ice pack to the area. Ice works as an anti-inflammatory, relieves muscle spasms, and acts as a painkiller. (Heat, on the other hand, addresses only the spasms.) A bag of frozen peas makes an excellent, flexible ice pack that adjusts easily to the shape of whatever body part you need it for. Wrap the bag in a pillowcase, and apply it to the affected area for ten to fifteen minutes. Watch to see that your skin doesn't turn red, which indicates that the ice has "burned" your skin and given you frost-

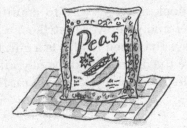

bite. (I have found that a pillowcase is most effective in preventing burns from frostbite.)

Mild discomfort is no cause for concern. But you should stop doing any exercise that causes pain to radiate down your arm or leg. Consult with your physician or a physical therapist about any pain that worsens, pain that persists for two weeks or more, or pain that radiates down an arm or leg. You may have a condition that requires medical intervention.

Besides radiating pain, symptoms that should be checked by a medical practitioner include:

- Unrelenting pain
- Pain that wakes you up at night
- Swelling or redness around an area
- Numbness and/or severe weakness in hands or feet
- Any pain that persists for longer than two weeks

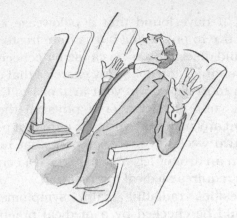

2. Brill Dead Chicken

In this version you'll be getting an extra neck stretch, which will counteract the protruded and bent-over positions in which we often hold our heads.

- Tuck in your chin and pull your head back, elongating the back of your neck.
- Push out your chest and lift it, pinching your shoulder blades together behind you.
- Bend your arms and pull your hands back toward your shoulders, keeping your elbows close to your torso and your palms facing outward.
- With your head still pulled back, tilt it backward until your face is parallel to the ceiling. Hold for a count of ten, and release.

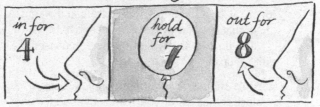

Nasal Breathing Rocks...

in for **4**

hold for **7**

out for **8**

Take a Deep Breath and Feel Better Fast

Even before you begin these exercises, you can give yourself the gift of a big, deep breath that will instantly relax you. When that happens, you will be able to listen better and pay more attention to what you are doing because your cells will be getting the oxygen they need to function optimally. (If you've ever found that pain disappears after aerobic exercise, here's why: when an activity causes your heart to pump more blood throughout your body, you increase your oxygen uptake, and oxygen helps every cell in the body function.)

And remember to breathe through your nose. Here's an easy reminder. I always say to patients, "You don't eat with your nose; therefore don't breathe with your mouth." There are practical reasons for nasal breathing. The nose filters and warms air so that your lungs are more receptive to it.

Just do the following any time you need a quick relaxer.

- While sitting down or lying on your back, place the palms of your hands over your stomach.

- Inhale deeply through your nostrils as you silently count to four. Feel your stomach inflate against your hands.

- Hold the breath as you silently count to seven.

- Exhale through your nostrils as you count to eight. You'll feel your hands move inward as your stomach deflates.

Author's Note

Always begin the exercises in a given chapter by doing the first exercise for each position—standing, sitting, or lying down. The reason is this: I always start with the exercise that I've found to be the most effective for the largest number of patients.

If doing that first exercise doesn't give you immediate relief, then go on to the next one. In fact, there is no harm in doing every Brill exercise in a chapter. Doing them all will help strengthen the problem area that much faster. And that means less pain in the future.

For variety's sake, I've written the directions explaining how to do some of the exercises on the right side of the body, and other exercises on the left side of the body, but you should of course adapt the instructions so that you do the exercise on whichever side has the ache or pain. Keep in mind, however, that most of the Brill exercises can benefit both sides of the body. So even if only one side hurts, you may want to perform the exercises on the opposite side as well; doing so will give you a comparison and will also give you an extra boost by helping to prevent future injury.

chapter 1

Your Head

If you are one of the millions of Americans prone to being sidelined by crippling headaches, it's time for a change. Although most people think that headaches are a normal and inevitable result of stress, headaches need *not* be the norm for you. I have a number of quick treatment options that have made most of my patients' stress-related headaches disappear fast—and they can do the same for you.

Using the simple techniques in this book, you will be able to take control and relieve headaches once you feel their symptoms coming on. There's no need to wait thirty minutes for an over-the-counter medication to kick in when you can get *Instant Relief* without any medication at all.

My techniques work because they are based on an understanding of the way stress affects the muscles that support the head, causing mechanical headaches. When you're under stress, you tend to tighten the muscles in the neck, skull, and face. These tight muscles can cause both vascular compression and nerve compression. Vascular compression means that blood vessels are being squeezed and can't deliver adequate oxygen to cells. Nerve compression results in less-than-optimum electrical-impulse delivery to muscles and inhibits muscular function.

Emotional stress, however, is not the only reason for mechanical headaches. The tight muscles that lead to so-called "mechanical headaches" also occur when you spend too long a time in a posture that forces your head out of what we call its neutral position. In the neutral position the head sits directly atop the neck in an alignment of relaxed verticality, which follows the gentle S shape of the entire spine with its curves at the neck, upper back, and lower back. If it remains in this position, the head will be well supported by all the vertebrae immediately below it—the vertebrae of the neck (the cervical spine) and the upper back (the thoracic spine), as well as the lumbar and sacral vertebrae—and also by the muscles and ligaments that connect to these vertebrae. The head needs all the support it can get, because it weighs between ten and twelve pounds—the weight of a bowling ball.

Unfortunately, your head is likely to spend much of its time without adequate support, because you put it into postures that take it out of neutral. If you spend a lot of time on the phone, for example, with your head tilted to hold the phone between your ear and your shoulder ("phone hugging"), you're forcing your head out of neutral position. If you spend a lot of time with your head in a protruded position, with the ears far forward of the shoulders—a position assumed by millions of people every day as they stare at their computer screens or bend over their paperwork—the head doesn't get the support it needs. Any posture that takes your head out of neutral position for an extended period of time has the potential to cause a headache because of the muscle tightening that occurs, and the vascular and nerve compression that result from muscle tightening.

There's another kind of nerve compression that can also result in a headache. Several of the twelve *cranial nerves*, which originate in the brain and are responsible for many functions, including the special senses of sight, hearing, smelling, and taste, pass through small openings at the base of the skull. If those nerves get compressed because of deviations in the head's normal position, they, too, can cause headaches.

Relieving your headache, however, may not be as simple as returning your head to its neutral position. If the head has remained in a protruded position for an extended period of time, bringing it back to neutral can stretch tight tissues, which leads to that common achiness at the back of the head, or above the ear or the eye on one side of the head. Even the scalp can become tense and cause discomfort. That's why I've provided a Brill exercise called a Scalp Glide (Exercise 7), which releases scalp tension.

Headaches are not the only problem to result from poor alignment. It can potentially cause long-term damage, too, because when the head spends much of its time in a protruded position, you are creating a situation that is like adding a hundred pounds of force on the vertebrae that support the head. This force compresses the disks between the vertebrae of the lower neck, as well as causing excessive wear and tear on the topmost vertebra (the atlas). If you don't balance these distortions of the head's natural alignment with movements in the opposite direction, you may experience early degeneration of the spine. Doing the Brill exercises will help prevent long-term damage.

The major focus of the Brill exercises, however, is on immediate pain relief. Most of the exercises I suggest for headaches emphasize sustaining a position that stretches the muscles of the upper neck and balances the out-of-neutral postures in which we spend so much of our time. By relieving compression in the upper neck, they help restore maximum blood flow and nerve function, which I've found to be the most effective way to relieve headaches quickly. But sometimes that kind of stretching doesn't work, and you're more likely to get relief if you tighten the already-tight muscles even more, holding your head in the extreme protruded position until the muscles finally relax. (See Exercise 12, Prone Neck Protrusion/Retraction, which does both.) It seems illogical, but it can be quite effective.

So try the Brill exercises, and see which ones work best for you. Don't let a headache overtake you—knock it out fast, and get on with your life.

Instant Relief for a Tension Headache

If, like so many millions of people, you clench your teeth or scowl when you're under stress, you probably get tension headaches, and you may feel pain or tightness in your jaw as well.

Here are several fast exercises that can relax the clenching and scowling motion and can be done whether you are sitting, standing, or lying down. Other exercises in this chapter work directly on the muscles of the eyes, the scalp, and the sinuses, another source of headache.

3. Tongue Press

The jaw, which works like a hinge, is able to open and close thanks to the muscles of the jaw. These muscles attach to the sides of the upper vertebrae in the neck, which are located just behind the ears. When those muscles become imbalanced—from sleeping on one side or from an altered bite, which could be caused by a broken crown, an unevenly filled tooth, teeth grinding, or even nail biting—you'll feel the impact in your jaw.

This nifty movement helps the jaw muscles by employing the tongue as a spring to align the hinges of the jaw so that they open and close normally, thus retraining the muscles to work symmetrically.

- Sit or stand up straight with your head facing forward, or lie on your back with your face toward the ceiling.
- Relax your jaw and mouth.
- Push the tip of your tongue against the roof of your mouth behind your upper teeth.
- Open and close your mouth, with your tongue against the roof of your mouth, ten times.

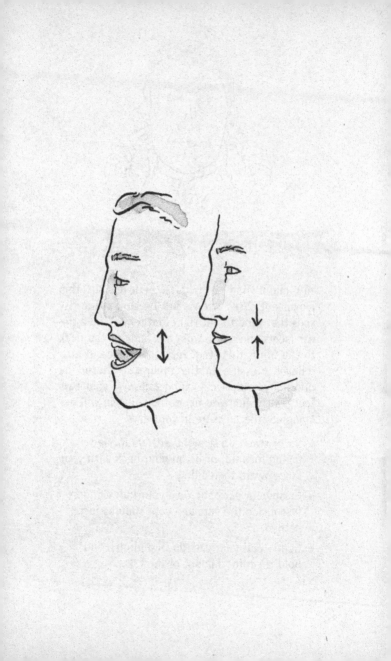

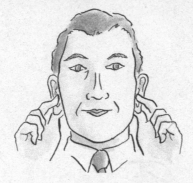

4. Ear Tug

You might find it hard to believe, but this movement eases a tense jaw by elongating tissues that tend to get tight and tense where the ear meets the neck. From the back of the neck to the front, this "tug" relaxes muscles. It also relieves pressure in the inner ear caused by grinding teeth or clenching a jaw. If your ears feel "full" when you fly, doing this tug will decompress the pressure in your ears.

- Sit or stand up straight with your head facing forward, or lie on your back with your face toward the ceiling.

- Grasp your earlobes with your index fingers just inside the ears and your thumbs just behind.

- Gently pull your ears down and out, and hold them for a count of ten.

If you grind your teeth or are prone to sinus headaches or jaw tension, doing this movement will relax the buccinator muscles, the sucking muscles in your cheeks, which keep the food between your teeth as you chew. As you do it, you may be reminded of that "face" you made behind someone's back when you were in school. But now you can put it to more practical use.

- Sit or stand up straight with your head facing forward, or lie on your back with your face toward the ceiling.
- Place your index fingers inside your cheeks.
- Gently pull your cheeks outward without straining your lips, and take a deep breath. Slowly exhale as you silently count to ten.

5. Cheek Release

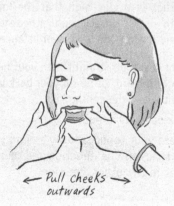

← Pull cheeks →
outwards

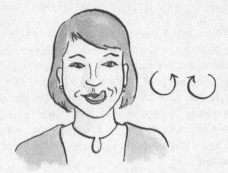

6. Tongue Loop

If your voice cracks and lowers when you get nervous, try this exercise, which rebalances the muscles attached to the tongue, as well as the muscles in the front of the neck that support the tongue and therefore affect how you speak.

When you do this Brill exercise the first time, you might find that it's easier to do in one direction. That is a sure sign that the length and strength of the muscles on either side of the neck and the tongue are out of balance.

- Sit or stand up straight with your head facing forward, or lie on your back with your face toward the ceiling.
- Stick out your tongue.
- Rotate your tongue slowly around your lips five times in one direction and then five times in the other direction.

Here's a way to release tension in the connective tissue between muscles in the front and back of your scalp. When you frown, muscles in the back of your scalp tense. Doing this gliding motion stretches the muscles that extend from the forehead up into the scalp as well as those that extend from the back of the head up into the scalp.

- Sit or stand up straight with your head facing forward, or lie on your back with your face toward the ceiling.
- Place your palms at the top of your forehead with fingers touching the scalp on either side.
- Glide the flesh of your scalp back and forth over your skull with your hands. Repeat ten times.

7. Scalp Glide

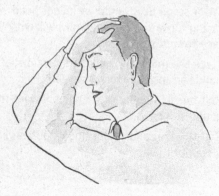

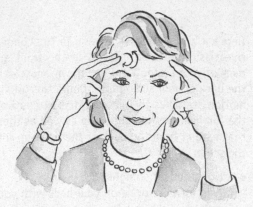

8. Forehead Roll

Not only will this movement relieve a tension headache, it's also great for easing eyestrain, draining clogged sinuses, and relieving forehead tension. If you spend long hours doing paperwork or logging in computer time, this one is for you.

- Sit or stand up straight with your head facing forward, or lie on your back with your face toward the ceiling.
- Place the index and middle fingers of both hands an inch above your eyebrows.
- Roll the skin under your fingers inward for a count of five.
- Roll the skin under your fingers outward for a count of five.

Eyestrain Relievers

To understand why you may be feeling eye-strain, think of your retinas as screens and your eye muscles as the focus mechanisms. The muscles are responsible for coordinating eye functions so that your vision can move from object to object.

But when you read for long periods of time with your eyes cast downward, for instance, you shorten and tighten certain eye muscles. Or if you have to look to one side to view your computer screen or protrude your neck in an attempt to get closer to it, these positions will weaken other eye muscles. That's why I always recommend setting up a computer where the screen is directly in front of you, an arm's length away. Placing papers on a slanted surface instead of flat in front of you will also help to balance eye muscles—while having the additional virtue of encouraging good posture.

In the meantime, if you've been attempting to read the fine print in tax forms, straining to look at your computer screen, or sitting through a one-day airing of a twelve-part TV series, try these eyestrain relievers. They will rebalance the five eye muscles you use to bring images to the retina efficiently.

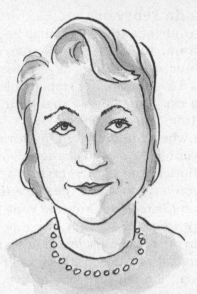

9. Eye Calisthenics (Straight)

- Sit or stand up straight with your head facing forward, or lie on your back with your face toward the ceiling.
- Roll your eyes up until you feel a slight ache in your eyes. Hold that position for a second or two. Then release your eyes to their normal position.
- Repeat the upward gaze and release five times.
- Close your eyes for the count of five.

- Sit or stand up straight with your head facing forward, or lie on your back with your face toward the ceiling.
- Look to the upper right and then to the lower left. Repeat five times.
- Look to the upper left and then to the lower right. Repeat five times.
- Put your hands together and rub them quickly until warm.
- Close your eyes, and place your warmed hands over them.
- Pull your eyes back into your head. (You'll feel them retract in their sockets.)
- Hold the position for a count of ten to let the eye muscles recover.

10. Eye Calisthenics (Diagonal)

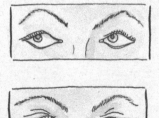

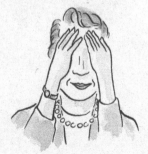

11. Sinus Drainer

Congested sinuses hurt, and they may make your head hurt, too. There are many different reasons why your four sinuses may become congested with mucus. The common cold is one culprit. Pollutants, irritants, pollen, dust mites, pet dander, mold, and mildew are other possible causes. To help your sinuses drain, try alternating five-minute applications of hot and cold compresses. Drinking hot water with lemon also helps to break up congestion. Avoid dairy foods and sugar, as they promote the formation of mucus.

If you suffer from sinus pain that worsens when you're under stress, try this:

- Sit or stand up straight with your head facing forward, or lie on your back with your face toward the ceiling.

- Place the index and middle fingers of each hand under your eyes and gently make circles toward the nose ten times.

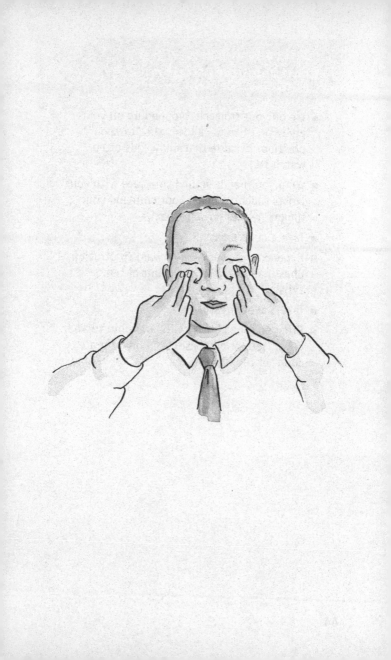

12. Prone Neck Protrusion/Retraction

- Lie on your stomach, propped up on your elbows. (I like to call this the "cartoon" position, because that's how kids often watch TV.)
- Wrap your hands around your face with your wrists touching under your chin and your fingers resting on your cheeks.
- Take a deep breath.
- Hyperextend your head forward (protrusion phase) and hold for the count of ten. Exhale.
- Take a deep breath.
- Bring your head back with your chin tucked down (retraction phase), and hold for a count of ten. Exhale.

Retraction Phase

Protrusion Phase

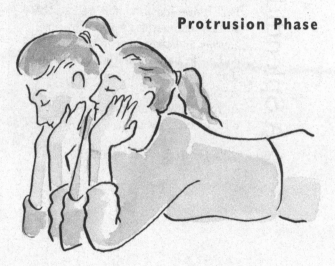

A Splendid Creation

The amazing human body has:

- 310 bones
- 650 muscles (more or less)
- 33 vertebrae
- 31 pairs of spinal nerves
- 2 cranial nerves
- 26 feet of intestine

Isn't it awe-inspiring how well all the parts work together? Most of the time, anyway. But they do need to work together, in balance and harmony, and that's what the exercises in this book are all about.

Your body is an absolutely divine gift. Tend to it wisely!

Your Neck

If stress strikes you in the neck, you have lots of company. That's probably why the expression "a pain in the neck" is part of our everyday language. If your neck is often so tight and tense that you can't turn or bend or lift your head without wincing, this section is specifically for you. But before giving you the Brill exercises for the neck, I have several common-sense do's and don'ts that will help. First, stop slouching. If you're in pain, sitting and standing straight can go a long way toward relieving the strain you're putting on your neck. Also, take frequent stretch breaks, especially if you put in long hours reading or working at the computer. And if you've been rotating your head in a full circular motion in order to relieve the pain, don't do it! This motion tends to compress the neck vertebrae, which will pinch nerves and irritate your neck even more. As for neck rubs, they offer only short-lived relief, if any. You need something more lasting.

The Brill neck exercises are proven movements specially designed to loosen that tightness and relieve your personal "pain in the neck" as soon as you feel it. They do so by helping to correct the misalignments of the neck that occur so frequently because of the natural flexibility of the structure of the neck.

The neck, built to perform eight different motions, is the most mobile part of the spine. The neck movements include:

- Flexion and extension (dropping the head forward and backward)
- Rotation (turning the head to the right and to the left)
- Side bends (dropping the head to the right and to the left)

The combined movements of the upper and lower neck allow other functional positions:

- Protraction (the upper neck extends as the lower neck flexes)
- Retraction (the upper neck flexes as the lower neck extends)

When the neck is aligned, the facet joints, which are the two contact points on each vertebra, and the disk, the third contact point, stay in proper balance. But because of the neck's great mobility, it's easy to get into unbalanced postures that can lead to discomfort and deformity. If you sit in a long, tense meeting with your neck stuck out in a protracted position, for example, you'll compress the vertebrae and the blood vessels that supply the vertebrae. During that meeting you may also tense your neck muscles—a response that often occurs when we're under stress—which will cause them to clamp down on the nerves within and interfere with their ability to deliver electrical impulses to the muscles. Either way, you will feel pain.

As a physical therapist, I evaluate the causes of a patient's neck pain, and its degree of seriousness, in order to classify it as one of three pain syndromes, each leading to the next if not corrected.

1. *Postural* pain stems from problems with how you sit, stand, and sleep. If it is not corrected, poor posture can lead to:
2. *Dysfunction* (pain and limited range of motion). This occurs when
   - A joint is stuck in a position and can't move out of it.
   - Spasms trigger muscular pain.
   - Scar tissue forms around a nerve root, triggering pain. (This is often the basis of carpal tunnel syndrome.)

If not treated, dysfunction can lead to:

3. *Derangement.* All derangements occur inside or around a joint. They include degenerative joint or disk disease; a cartilage, ligament, or muscle tear, or a disk that herniates—that is, bulges or prolapses—or even worse, ruptures, leaving fragmented pieces trapped between the nerve and the vertebrae.

To stop your needless suffering and relieve that neck pain, start doing the Brill exercises now. You'll see that I've included here a number of variations on the two Brill Chicken neck retractions (Exercises 1 and 2; see Introduction). Retraction restores balance to the neck muscles, aligns the vertebral disks, permits maximal blood circulation from the heart to the brain, and allows optimal flow of electricity through nerves to the organs and extremities—as evidenced by the instant recovery of strength you will experience when you do a retraction.

Exercises 13 to 18—all variations on the Brill Chicken exercises—operate on the same principles as Exercises 1 and 2.

The easiest retraction—the classic form—appears first because I've found that acute episodes of neck pain respond to it so well. The ones that follow increase in intensity and are particularly helpful for stiff necks and more chronic neck problems, especially ones that last longer than three months.

You don't have to wait until a sudden pain

hits to use these exercises to your advantage. Doing them throughout the day is an excellent way to prevent the neck strains caused by the stress of daily living. So let's get started on relieving—or, better yet, preventing—that neck pain.

13. Neck Retraction (Classic Form)

Doing this movement, and its variations, will decompress the nerves that come out of the skull, allowing them maximal delivery of their electrical impulses to the neck muscles. Neck retractions also restore normal length to the muscles of the neck, which often become short and tight because of poor posture.

- Sit or stand up straight with your head facing forward.
- Slide your head back, tucking your chin so that the back of your neck is elongated and your ears glide behind your shoulders. (The double chin that results is temporary.)
- Hold for a count of ten.

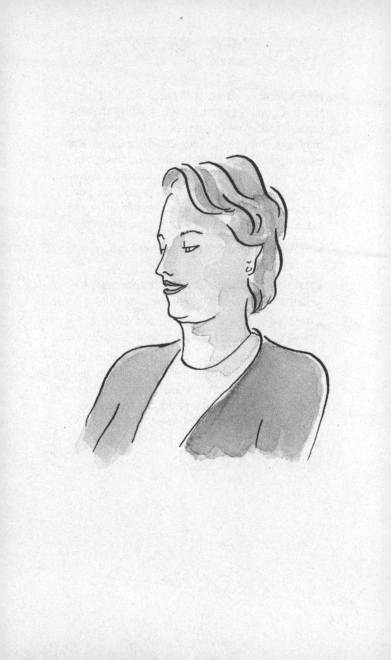

14. Towel Stretch

If you awaken with a stiff neck, this Brill exercise is a quick way to help you mobilize the vertebrae that are responsible for producing tightness throughout your upper shoulders and lower neck. The motion also helps to prevent osteoporosis and eliminate the unsightly dowager's hump that develops from chronically poor posture. You can do this exercise right after you get out of the shower.

- Stand up straight with your head facing forward.
- Take a bath towel, and fold it down about half an inch along one of the long sides.
- Grab each end of the towel, and drape it around the back of your neck, at its base.
- Slide your head back, tucking your chin so that the back of your neck is elongated and your ears glide behind your shoulders. Press your neck backward against the resistance of the towel as you pull the towel forward.
- Repeat ten times.

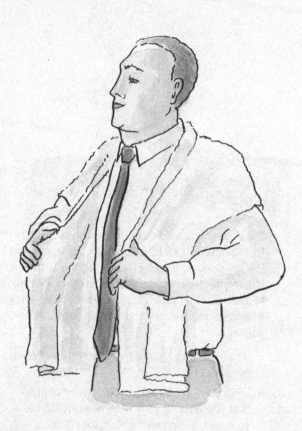

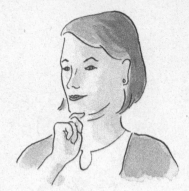

15. Neck Retraction with Chin Push

Using your fingers to create overpressure helps to promote full mobility of both the upper and the lower neck, thereby counteracting stiffness. When you have maximum upper-neck flexion, headaches will disappear; increasing lower-neck extension reduces disk herniation, which is very common.

- Sit or stand up straight with your head facing forward.
- Slide your head back, tucking your chin so that the back of your neck is elongated and your ears glide behind your shoulders.
- Push the index finger of one hand against your chin.
- Hold for a count of ten.

This easy movement concentrates on the lower part of the neck, an area often beset by dysfunction.

- Sit or stand up straight with your head facing forward.
- Clasp your hands together, and place them behind your head (not your neck).
- Tuck your chin, and push your head back against your hands for a count of ten.

16. Neck Retraction with Resistance

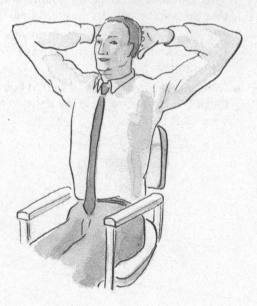

17. Neck Retraction with Extension

When you bend your head backward in this movement, you won't feel any dizziness if you emphasize the chest lift. That will help you avoid pinching the vertebral arteries, which make a 90-degree turn at the upper segments of both sides of your neck. If you experience dizziness anyway, stop doing the exercise immediately. Dizziness may be an indication of a problem that should be addressed by a physician.

- Sit or stand up straight with your head facing forward.
- Slide your head back, tucking your chin so that the back of your neck is elongated.
- Lift your chest, and as you do, bend your head backward. (Imagine your heart is lifting to the ceiling.)
- When you've lifted your head so that you're looking at the ceiling, hold the position for a count of ten.

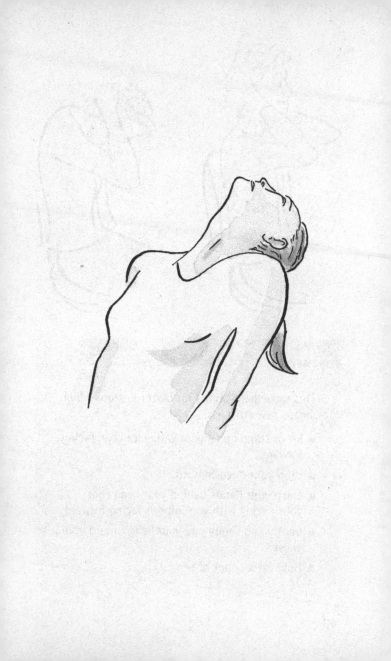

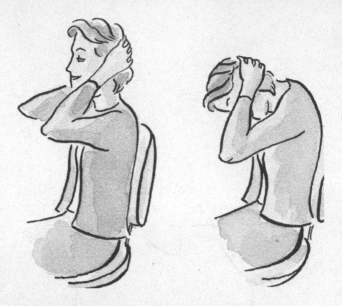

18. Neck Flexion

This movement allows for better flexion, which means less stiffness.

- Sit or stand up straight with your head facing forward.
- Drop your head forward.
- Clasp your hands behind your head (not your neck!) with your elbows facing forward.
- Gently and firmly pull your head toward your chest.
- Hold for a count of ten.

Neck Benders and Balancers

The ability to bend to the side and to rotate the neck from one side to the other is an important neck function. Try backing out of a driveway or parking space without adequate neck rotation—it's difficult and possibly dangerous. We rotate our necks hundreds of times a day without a thought—until one day pain hits. The overpressure in Exercises 19 and 20 allows for increased range of motion and will help to prevent pain.

The reason that these exercises have directions to "repeat on the left side" is to ensure that the neck muscles that work when you rotate your neck, or bend your head to your shoulders, will be evenly balanced. You will then have some protection against the damage done when you hold your neck in a sustained rotation, for example when you stare at a computer monitor off to one side of your desk. Such rotations can create neck imbalances that produce pain, premature degenerative processes, and scoliosis.

Strength Test

To appreciate the near-miraculous muscle-strengthening that results from doing a neck retraction, try this with a friend. Extend your right arm in front of you at shoulder height, and tell your friend to press down gently on your arm, then more and more firmly, until you can resist the pressure no longer and the arm goes down. Repeat on the left side, and determine which arm is stronger. Then do one of the neck retractions. After the neck retraction, repeat the arm strength test with your friend, on the weaker arm. See how much more strength you now have? These retractions make a world of difference in your upper-body strength.

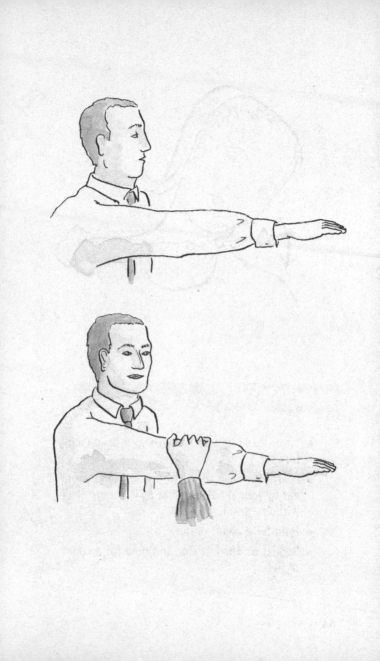

19. Side Neck Bends

- Sit or stand up straight with your head facing forward.
- Lean your head to the right, dropping your ear to your shoulder as far as it can go without straining.
- Hold for a count of five.
- Repeat on the left side and hold for a count of five.

- Sit up straight with your back against the chair.
- Grab the left side of the seat with your left hand.
- Tilt your head down to your right shoulder.
- Raise your right arm and place your hand on the left side of your head.
- Use the right hand to gently pull your head farther into the neck stretch.
- When your neck is stretched to the right as far as it can go without straining, hold the position for a count of five.
- Repeat on the left side and hold for a count of five.

20. Side Neck Bends with Overpressure

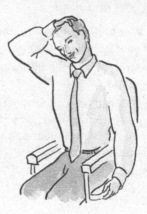

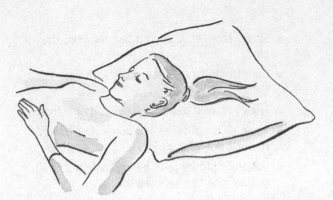

21. Neck Retraction on Pillow

If you wake up with a stiff neck, here's a quick way to relieve your discomfort. Placing the pillow as shown tilts your head, which allows you to retract your neck more.

- Lie on your back with a pillow under the top part of your head.
- Keep your head straight with your face looking upward.
- Press your head back against your pillow, tucking your chin so that the back of your neck is elongated and your ears glide behind your shoulders.
- Repeat ten times.

3

Your Shoulders

"Muscle guarding," a very common physiological reaction to stress, often takes the form of scrunching up your shoulders toward your ears. This reflexive attempt to protect yourself from harm creates a whole chain reaction in your neurological and orthopedic systems, frequently culminating in shoulder pain.

The *neurological* fact you need to know to understand your pain is that the nerves in the lower neck, and the eleventh cranial nerve, constitute all the nerves that supply the muscles supporting the shoulders. When muscle guarding causes the nerves in the neck to be compressed between the vertebrae, the nerves that go to the shoulders can't fire their electrical charges efficiently, and therefore the shoulder muscles, which work to keep the shoulder joint in alignment, can't function the way they should.

The *orthopedic* fact you need to know is that the extreme mobility of the shoulder joint—it is the most mobile joint in the body—makes it particularly vulnerable to problems of instability. So when the supporting muscles don't function properly, the shoulders are quick to suffer with pain, limited range of motion, and weakness.

But muscle guarding is only one of many challenges to the muscles that support the shoulder joint, and to the shoulder joint itself. Repetitive motions, like lifting a child, painting a ceiling, playing racquetball, or lifting weights, can cause the muscles at the front of the shoulder—especially the anterior deltoids, the biceps, and the major and minor pectorals—to tighten so that they dominate the shoulder motion, at the expense of the muscles that attach at the back of the shoulder, including the large trapezius and the latissimus dorsi. Even a less active pursuit, like spending hours moving a computer mouse with your arm extended too far in front of you or hugging a phone between your shoulder and your ear during a long conversation, can result in imbalances between the front and back muscles of the shoulder, altering the length/strength ratio that must exist between those muscles to assure proper joint movement.

When the muscles are out of balance, the shoulder joint can be thrown forward, off its axis of rotation, and it won't be able to glide, roll, and spin the way it's supposed to. This will affect the joint's ability to move the arm painlessly through its three planes of motion—extending and flexing, abducting and adducting, and rotating inwardly and outwardly.

The pain you feel when the muscles that support the shoulder don't do their job of moving the bones of the joint in a smooth and controlled manner is the result of the bones being out of alignment and rubbing against one or more of the other structures that are part of the joint—a tendon, a bursa, or the joint capsule itself. This is what we call impingement, and it causes an inflammatory response. So let me introduce you to *-itis*, the Latin suffix indicative of inflammation—as in *tendinitis*, *bursitis*, and *capsulitis*.

In the shoulder, as in every joint in the body, *tendons* attach muscle to bone. Made up of connective tissue similar to that of ligaments (which attach bone to bone and act as passive restraints to motion), tendons are more supple and pliable than ligaments. But unlike ligaments, which are not subject to inflammation, tendons can become inflamed; which happens when bones rub against them. If the resulting tendinitis persists, it can develop into bone spurs, callus-like structures that are visible on X rays.

The *bursas* are fluid-filled sacs found in many of the joints of the body. In the shoulder joint as elsewhere, they act as cushions between bone and fibrous tissue—facilitating the friction-free movement of the muscles and tendons as they pull on the bones. When the bursas are inflamed, the result is bursitis.

The shoulder *capsule* is made up of fibrocartilage, which protects the joint. Inflammation of that cartilage can result in adhesive capsulitis (also known as frozen shoulder), which creates severe limitations in the range of motion in the shoulder and greater and greater pain over time if not treated. It tends to affect women more than men and occurs for no apparent reason. But I have noticed a pattern of muscle imbalance in patients with adhesive capsulitis: their anterior (front) muscle group tends to be short and tight, and their posterior (back) muscle group tends to be weak.

What happens to the shoulder joint as a result of improperly balanced muscles is typical of the damage done to any joint in the body if the muscles that connect to and support it are pulling on it asymmetrically. The goal of the Brill exercises is to get the nerves that run from the neck through the shoulder muscles firing properly, the muscles rebalanced, and the joint returned to its normal axis of rotation. You will then experience pain-free movement of the shoulder through all its extraordinary range of motion.

The more you do the Brill exercises, the less likely you are to experience pain, and the more protection you'll be giving to your shoulder joints. Over the long term these exercises can also help you to avoid the onset of a degenerative joint disease like arthritis and the formation of bone spurs.

The next time that stress or anxiety or fear forces you into muscle guarding, or you're suffering the effects of repetitive motion or of sustained out-of-alignment shoulder positions, you'll know what to do for instant relief. So start doing the Brill exercises—now.

Balance Is All

Before doing one or more of my tension-relievers to remedy pain or tension in your shoulders, here's a suggestion that may ultimately make them unnecessary for some of you: balance all the stuff you carry around evenly. If you are one of those people who weigh themselves down with multiple loads—with tote bags, laptop computers, briefcases, purses, suitcases—either carry them in two hands, *or* sling them over both shoulders. Don't carry one bag with your right hand and hang another one over your left shoulder. Remember all those times when you walked tipped to one side, like a human Tower of Pisa? One shoulder is going to suffer. But it doesn't have to. Balance and equalize what you're hauling—your shoulders will thank you for it.

Alternatively, if you are one of the rare people who carry only one item at a time, balance your load by switching it every day so that one side doesn't suffer from overuse. For example, if you tend to sling a pocketbook over your right shoulder all the time, start to alternate with your left shoulder.

Other tips for minimizing pain in the shoulders: alternate which side you lie on when you sleep, and avoid sleeping on your belly or with your arm over your head.

Finally, if you lift weights, follow the tips for injury-free workouts for the upper body in *The Core Program*. They will help you avoid the common pitfall of overdeveloping your already dominant muscles, while neglecting the muscles necessary for good postural alignment.

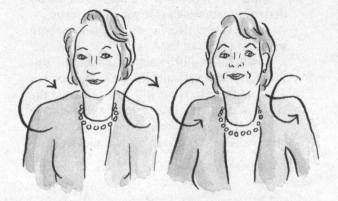

22. Backward Shoulder Circles

These backward shoulder circles counteract the dominant front muscle group, the pectorals, biceps, and anterior deltoids, which constantly pull the shoulders forward.

- Pull your shoulders up.
- Rotate them to the back.
- Drop them down, pinching the shoulder blades together.
- Circle them forward.
- Repeat as a continuous motion ten times.

- Raise your right arm out in front of you at shoulder level.
- Move your arm to the left so that it is across your chest as far as it can go.
- Move your left arm underneath the right, and place your left hand on your right upper arm.
- Pull the right arm to the left and hold for a count of ten.
- Repeat with the left arm.

23. Cross Chest

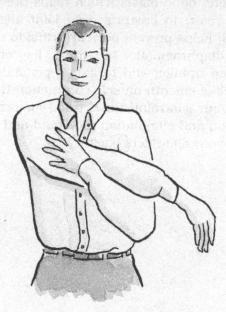

Tight Pecs

Hunching repeatedly over a work surface, whether it's a desk, a stove, or a home repair project, can cause the pectoral muscles to become shortened and tight. This in turn can pull the shoulder joints out of alignment. Exercises 24 to 27 will enable you to elongate your pectorals to their functional length, which will help alleviate pain in the short run and help prevent problems that result from misaligned shoulder joints in the long run.

Elongating your pectoral muscles also allows you to pull your shoulders back and assume good posture. Good posture is critical to building bone mass, which helps prevent osteoporosis; to creating good joint alignment, which helps prevent osteoarthritis; to promoting diaphragmatic breathing for optimum oxygen uptake; and to aiding peristalsis (the wavelike smooth muscle contraction throughout your gastrointestinal tract) for proper digestion and elimination. So stand and sit tall, with your shoulders back.

With this exercise you'll get instant relief from the shoulder pain that often results from tight pecs.

- Stand in a doorway with your feet shoulder-width apart. Extend your right foot about six inches in front of the doorway.

- Raise your right arm to a 90-degree angle from the side of your torso, bend your elbow, and place your forearm, from elbow to palm, flat against the door frame.

- Slightly turn your body away from the arm until you feel a stretch in your pectorals. Hold for a count of ten.

- Repeat with the left arm.

24. Doorway Pectoral Stretch at 90 Degrees

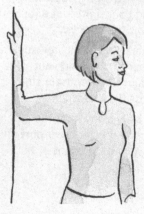
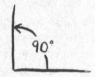

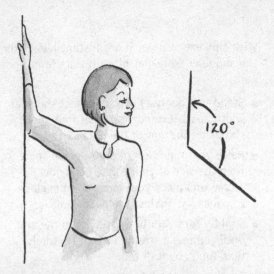

25. Doorway Pectoral Stretch at 120 Degrees

- Stand in a doorway with your feet shoulder-width apart. Extend your right foot about six inches in front of the doorway.

- Raise your right arm to a 120-degree angle from the side of your torso, bend your elbow, and place your forearm, from elbow to palm, flat against the door frame.

- Slightly turn your body away from the arm until you feel a stretch in the lower portion of your pectorals. Hold for a count of ten.

- Repeat with the left arm.

Give yourself a "lift" with this nifty stretch.

- Clasp your hands behind your back.
- Lift up your chest.
- With your hands still clasped, lift up your arms as far as you can, maintaining an upright position. Hold for a count of ten.

26. Hands Behind Back Pectoral Stretch (Seated)

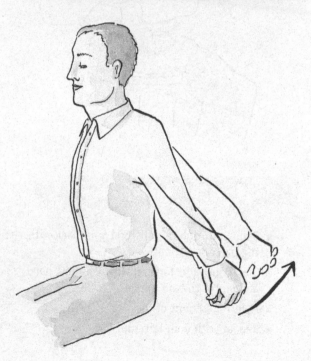

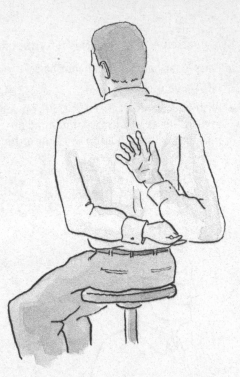

27. Arm Pull Behind Back

- Bend your right arm behind your back with the palm facing outward.
- Grab your right forearm with your left hand, and pull it toward the left.
- Hold for a count of ten.
- Repeat with your left arm.

Here's another good exercise to relieve shoulder pain. With this movement you are using the weight of your arm to "distract" the shoulder joint—that is, to create spaces in the joint—in order to relieve cartilage impingement from the pressure created by the weight of one bone pressing against another. Often prescribed after shoulder surgery, it's a gentle way to give range of motion to an injured shoulder.

- Lean on a desk or the back of a chair on the uninjured side.
- Let the other arm dangle down with the thumb facing outward.
- Swing the dangling arm clockwise in small circles five times, then swing it counterclockwise five times.

28. Pendulums

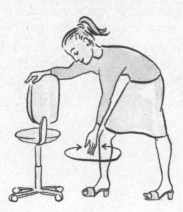

29. Brill Prone Chicken

The Brill Chicken elongates tightened pectorals, strengthens the upper-back muscles that control the shoulder blades, and stretches the neck muscles to decompress lower-neck segments. As you saw in the Introduction, you can do the Brill Chicken either sitting or standing, which will give you a great stretch. In this lying-down variation you are also stretching your pectorals while you are strengthening your upper back through resisting gravity. This will result in greater back strength and better posture when you sit upright.

- Lie on your stomach.
- Tuck in your chin and pull your head back to elongate the back of your neck.
- Push out your chest and pinch your shoulder blades together.
- Bend your arms, keeping the elbows close to your torso with your wrists pulled back, and the palms facing away from your head.
- Raise your head, chest, and arms off the floor or bed, hold for a count of ten, and gently release.

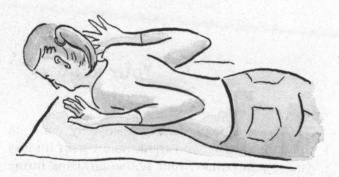

chapter 4

Your Elbows

Maybe elbows don't immediately come to mind when you think about pain (unless you've just banged your not-so-amusing funny bone). If so, it's time to look at these joints in a different way, because they are actually potential sources of a number of problems that manifest in other parts of the body and can affect your everyday activities. For example, if shaking hands or grasping an object results in sudden pain, that's a pretty clear indication that your elbow joint is involved. Depending on its severity, the pain may limit your ability to grip objects, from holding a pen to lifting a tennis racket. These actions may even become impossible.

The cause can be traced to the three nerves

of the hand—the *radial,* the *median,* and the *ulnar*—that are terminal branches of the *brachial plexus,* which supplies all the nerves to the upper extremities. These nerves run through the elbow, providing sensory input, including sensations of pain, touch, heat, and cold, to the forearms and hands, and delivering electrical impulses to the muscles that control movement in those parts of the body.

Lying close to the skin's surface, these nerves lack the protection of fatty tissue. So they can easily be pinched during one of the many routine activities often performed with the forearms leaning against the sharp edge of a table or desk for a prolonged period of time—such activities as typing, writing, or sewing, for example. Pressure on those nerves means that your hands are going to suffer.

The radial nerve runs along the forearm on the thumb side. It serves the muscles that extend into the elbow, wrist, and thumb. Pain or weakness along the muscles at these sites indicates radial nerve involvement. The problem can come from anywhere along the nerve pathway, from the neck to the thumb.

The median nerve supplies the forearm flexors as well as the five muscles of the hand. It passes through the tunnel between the eight carpal bones and the soft tissues in the wrist. Weakness in the index and middle fingers, and the inner part of the thumb as well as the hand, indicates median nerve involvement. Grip strength is compromised.

The ulnar nerve loops through the crease under the elbow, near the surface of the skin and into the hand. The "funny bone" pain conveyor, it passes down the arm on the pinkie side. A weak pinkie suggests ulnar nerve entrapment somewhere along the nerve's path.

Nerve entrapment, or compression, is a frequent problem for the radial, median, and ulnar nerves, because there are so many activities—such as talking on the phone with your shoulder scrunched up to your ear, typing for long periods of time, not to mention whiplash—that can result in the scarring and inflammation of the nerve sheaths that cause the compression. To make sure that these nerves aren't compressed, I've provided a series of Brill exercises called "nerve glides." These movements glide the nerves through the sheaths that surround them. Think of a nerve as a string that runs through a straw without touching the sides. The nerve itself has no flexibility and can't be stretched, but the sheath surrounding it does have flexibility, because it contains elastin and collagen. The gliding movement helps to stretch the sheath.

The combined effect of the glide and the stretch is to release the nerve from any kind of adherence that causes it to stick to the sheath, including any scar tissue that may have formed from an injury. By freeing the nerve, the glide enables it to transmit full electrical power to the muscles. The muscles around the nerve will then work the way they should. And, because blood vessels are in close proximity to nerves, the nerve glides will improve circulation, too.

Nerve glides are excellent techniques to rid your hands of pain, tingling, and weakness. At the same time they will help your elbow joints to move more freely so that you can extend and flex, rotate your forearms, and even hit a tennis or golf ball without elbow pain. The next time your elbow hurts, turn to these Brill exercises for fast relief.

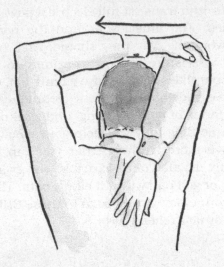

30. Triceps Muscle Stretch

The triceps are the primary extenders of the elbow and the shoulder, so give them this good stretch, which will help relieve elbow pain.

- Raise your right arm straight up next to your right ear.
- Bend the elbow and rest your right palm on your back.
- Cup your left hand around your right elbow.
- Pull the right elbow toward the left as far as possible. Hold for a count of ten.
- Repeat with your left arm.

Nerve Sheath Stretches

Exercises 31 to 33 will help the ulnar, median, and radial nerves by stretching the surrounding sheaths. This frees them to glide right through those sheaths, which will restore strength to the hands, help blood circulation, and relieve "pins and needles" sensations.

This movement looks weird, but it does help relieve pressure on the ulnar nerves.

- Make O's with the thumbs and index fingers of each hand.
- Turn your hands upside down and place the O's over your eyes.
- Place the other fingers on your cheeks, and push your elbows back as far as you can while your hands remain on your face. Hold for a count of ten.

31. Ulnar Nerve Glide (Birdman)

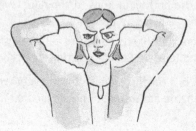

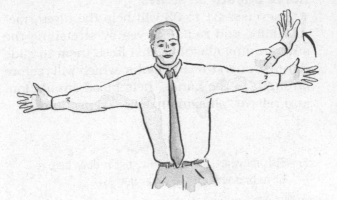

32. Median Nerve Glide (The Carpal Tunnel Reliever)

Inflammation and scarring of the median nerve contribute to the tingling, weakness, and pain in the hands known as carpal tunnel syndrome. The rapid movements of this exercise will glide the median nerve through the soft tissues surrounding it.

- Raise both your arms to shoulder level with the palms facing forward.
- Flex your hands backward as far as you can and release. Repeat ten times quickly.

This is a terrific exercise to do every two hours when you are working on a keyboard.

- Raise your arms to shoulder level with the palms facing backward.
- Make fists with your thumbs inside the other fingers.
- Flex your wrists back and forth ten times quickly.

33. Radial Nerve Glide

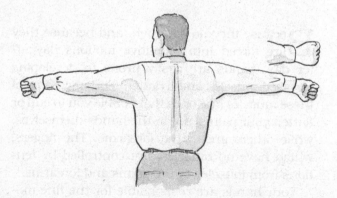

Your Hands

Because they do so much, and because they are forced into repetitive motions day after day, hands are easily prone to developing stressed muscles and irritated tendons. Some of these muscles (the ones that enable you to cup or flatten your palms) are in the hands themselves, while others are in the forearms. The fingers, which have no muscles, are controlled by tendons from muscles in the palms and forearms.

Your hands are responsible for the fine motor control necessary to perform all kinds of tasks that require precision. So a sudden pain in a hand is more than a discomfort; it can be a real hindrance. When pain strikes, everything you do with your hands, from cutting vegetables to lifting a toddler, from typing at your computer to playing a musical instrument, from holding on to the steering wheel to sewing on a button, becomes difficult.

The widespread use of computers is a real culprit in hand pain. Unlike typewriters, which gave you a chance to extend your hands when you had to stop to return the carriage or fix a mistake with a correct strip, computers don't offer built-in breaks. Not only that: typewriters featured spring-loaded keys, which provided some give when the fingertips hit them; but computer keyboards are hard-loaded, delivering repeated small blows to the fingertips as they tap the keys. Spending too much time with the fingers bent over the keys will also overwork the muscles that close the hand, making them tight and short, while weakening the underused muscles that open the hand. Laptops are particularly bad offenders because they force hands into very cramped positions for extended periods of time.

Your hands are no different from any other part of your body: stress one muscle group over another, and the joint between them will be pulled out of its correct position. When that happens, you're going to feel pain and lose mobility and strength. Eventually the joints of your fingers may take on the crooked, gnarled appearance that is so often seen in aging hands and is assumed to be an inevitable part of old age. But that deformity is actually the result of repetitive strains that have altered the balance of the muscles pulling on delicate joint structures. If it remains untreated, the resulting imbalance can progress to arthritis. However, there's a lot you can do to slow or halt that process.

As a physical therapist, I always treat the cause, not the symptoms. To treat as well as to prevent hand problems, I prescribe exercises to strengthen the muscles that open the hands. By keeping these muscles strong and active, these Brill exercises also help lubricate the joints with synovial fluid, which is produced when the cartilage that covers the bony surface of each joint is stimulated by the movement of the joint.

As a general principle, you should remember to frequently stretch your hands in the direction opposite to any position they have remained in for an extended period of time. This will help restore muscular balance and pull your joints into normal alignment.

You can also take some very simple steps to protect your hands. For instance, buy utensils with bigger handles. You won't be forced to grip them so hard, preventing the stressing of muscles. Push a pen or pencil through the foam of a hair curler—your fingers will be cushioned when you write. When you lift weights, wear gloves for a firmer contact without having to grip the weights so tightly—just rest the weights in relaxed hands.

These Brill exercises may extend the longevity of your healthy hands while giving you instant relief. So take care of your hands! They are the best tools you'll ever have.

And remember: even if the instructions explain how to do an exercise on the right side, or tell you to do it "on the side that hurts," doing it on both sides can only be beneficial. That way you'll get pain relief now, and prevent pain in the future.

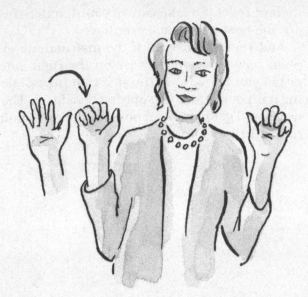

34. Finger Flexion

This exercise and the next one will relieve finger pain, and ease stiffness throughout your hands.

- Lift your hands.
- Bend the fingers of both hands down simultaneously so that the tips of the fingers reach the knuckle pads of the palms. Your thumbs should be relaxed.
- Repeat ten times.

- Lift your right arm straight out in front of you, palm facing upward.
- Using your left hand, pull the fingers of your right hand back. Hold for a count of ten.
- Repeat on the left side.

35. Palm Stretch with Finger Extension

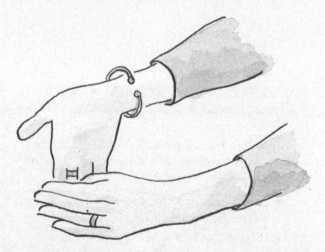

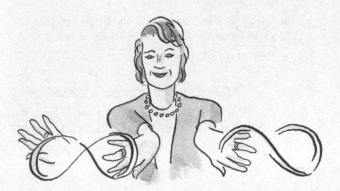

36. Figure 8's

This fluid motion promotes blood circulation, decreases swelling, and restores full range of motion to the wrist.

- Extend your arms straight out in front of you below shoulder level.
- Let your hands drop below your wrists, and move them through figure-8 rotations ten times.

If you've been experiencing pain in your wrist, this Brill exercise will create an opening between the wrist bones and relieve pressure within the carpal tunnel, through which the median nerve passes.

- Grasp the wrist that hurts between the middle finger and the thumb of the other hand.
- Keeping the forearm motionless, pull the wrist away from the forearm, and hold for a count of ten.

37. Wrist Distraction

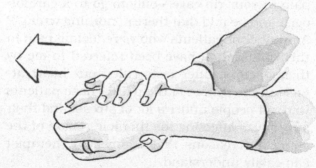

chapter

6

Your Mid-Back

Have you ever thought you were having a heart attack because you felt a stabbing pain in your rib cage—only to go to a cardiologist and be told that there's "nothing wrong"? A number of patients who were feeling pain in their midsection have been referred to me by their doctors, after tests ruled out heart attack as the source of the pain. These patients were all people under a lot of stress, and their stress was affecting the thoracic region of the spine, for reasons that a physical therapist can easily understand.

No one should simply assume that such pain is stress-related, but if your doctor has given your heart a clean bill of health and

Know the Symptoms of a Heart Attack

Conventional thinking notwithstanding, heart disease is the number-one killer of both women and men. Although women may experience the same symptoms as men when they have a heart attack, often the warning signs present differently, and are harder to distinguish from everyday aches and pains. But one way to distinguish them is by circumstance, since in women these symptoms are often brought on by exertion. Seek medical attention immediately if you experience these symptoms:

Men

Crushing chest pain

Shortness of breath

Women

Burning sensation or pressure in the chest

Arm pain

Pain between shoulder blades

Upper abdominal pain

Flu-like symptoms, including fatigue, dizziness, and nausea

you are still getting that pain, this chapter is for you.

The *thoracic spine*—that area between the neck and the abdomen—contains twelve thoracic vertebrae. Each of these vertebrae attaches to two ribs—one on either side of the body. There are twelve of these pairs of ribs. Ten of the twelve rib pairs wrap around the front of the body and attach to the *sternum,* or chest bone. Muscles in the thoracic spine attach up from the pelvis and down from the neck. The anatomy of the thoracic area enables it to serve as the most stable part of the spine, a solid central core area anchoring the more mobile neck and lumbar spine.

The thoracic spine also assists the motion of, and gives stability to, the shoulder complex. Anytime you reach up or out from your shoulder, the thoracic spine has to be able to rotate, extend, and flex.

One of the things we do when we are stressed is to hunch our shoulders and round our mid-backs. These "guarding" postures are a reflexive attempt to protect ourselves, an unconscious physical response to a psychological stress.

Unfortunately, when our shoulders tense and pull forward and our chests cave in, the muscles between and surrounding the rib cage can't function at their maximal capacity. One possible result may be *costochondritis,* an inflammatory process involving the muscles and tendons that attach to the ribs and sternum, which can cause either an achy or a stabbing chest pain. Costochondritis occurs because the pectoral muscles and the intercostal muscles between the ribs get tight from overuse when we hunch over for extended periods of time.

If you don't have adequate postural strength in your upper back, you may also develop costochondritis from doing repetitive push-ups, lifting a child over and over again, or even from spending hours using a computer mouse. The pain of costochondritis can also occur when poor posture shifts a rib out of position so that the rib impinges on nerves that pass between it and an adjacent rib.

In addition to its stabilizing and mobilizing capacities, the thoracic spine performs a unique function: it protects the heart, the lungs, and the diaphragm, the primary respiratory muscle. The diaphragm is a domelike muscle that sits underneath the rib cage. When you inhale, your diaphragm expands downward, making the abdomen protrude. When you exhale, it rises up to deflate the lungs. Unfortunately, another consequence of sitting in a rounded-in position is diminished lung capacity, because the diaphragm doesn't have enough room to work properly.

If you are under stress, I advise you to take at least one deep breath every hour. Doing so will give you renewed energy, release tension you didn't even know you were holding in, and allow your shoulders to descend to a relaxed position.

So go ahead now and inhale for four seconds, hold your breath for seven seconds, and exhale for eight seconds. Exhaling twice as long as inhaling forces all the carbon dioxide out of your lungs, making room for more oxygen to come in. Every cell of your body responds well to oxygen. Deep breathing also causes full expansion of the lungs, both horizontally and vertically, so that the intercostals, which are also important respiratory muscles, expand and contract, becoming more efficient.

To combat stress-related pain, all the Brill exercises in this chapter are geared toward moving the thoracic spine through its optimal range of motion—that is, flexion, extension, side bends, and rotation. These motions, as they pump blood through your muscles and joints, will ensure that proper posture and a healthy spine are yours, and they will go a long way toward eradicating stress-induced pain. By keeping your thoracic spine mobile, these exercises will also protect your cervical and lumbar spine, which have to compensate by moving excessively if the thoracic area becomes too stiff.

Scoliosis: A Curvature in the Mid-Back

Constantly rotating your spine in one direction when you sit at your desk can cause *scoliosis*, a condition in which the spine curves to one side and makes you lopsided. I've seen this happen in many patients whose computer is at an angle to where they sit instead of directly in front of them, for example. But this is only one of the many musculoskeletal imbalances that commonly result in scoliosis. Most cases of scoliosis can be traced to muscular imbalances either above or below the area of curvature, which the thoracic spine—the midspine area—tries to compensate for. The compensation is part of the sensory system's balancing act, the main goal of which is to keep your head, specifically your eyes and ears, on a level, rather than tilted, plane. But when there are inequalities of strength in muscle groups that oppose one another in the areas above and below the thoracic spine, your midback pays the price of this balancing act. The resulting curvature can impede spinal motion and rib cage expansion; if the curvature becomes more severe, it can diminish lung capacity and interfere with digestive functions.

All the exercises that follow will help correct the muscle imbalances that constitute nineteen out of the twenty causes of scoliosis. (The twentieth cause, a congenital abnormality, can only be corrected by surgery.)

Exercises 38 to 42 maximize the efficiency of the rib cage and the thoracic spine by opening, closing, and rotating the ribs and vertebrae in the area.

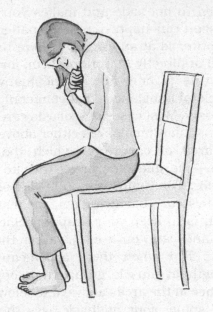

38. Hug Yourself

This first stretch opens both the thoracic spine and the ribs, thereby relieving tightness and allowing optimal expansion of the respiratory muscles, which will result in better breathing.

- Wrap your arms around your body.
- Round your back, allowing your head to drop forward.
- Hold the position for a count of ten.

This motion closes the spaces between the ribs and between the vertebrae of the thoracic spine, thereby allowing the thoracic spine to extend for functions you do daily, like lifting your arms or throwing.

- Bend your elbows over your head, keeping your palms and wrists pressed against each other and your elbows as close together as possible.
- Lift your chest and your arms until you feel a stretch in your mid-back.
- Hold the position for a count of ten.

Follow this movement with Exercise 40, Be a Genie, for an optimal mid-back stretch.

39. Seated Backward Bend

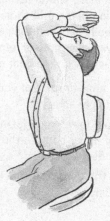

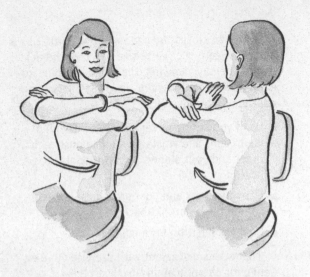

40. Be a Genie

Doing this exercise while sitting will accentuate the rotation in the mid-thoracic region (the part of your body between the neck and the abdomen). If you play golf or tennis, this rotational movement will help your game.

- Cross your arms in front of your chest, and grab your upper arms.
- Keeping your lower body facing forward, rotate your upper body to the right. Hold for a count of five.
- Repeat in the opposite direction. Hold for a count of five.

Slouching tightens the muscles between the ribs and pelvis. This stretch opens the rib cage as well as the muscles that attach to them.

- Sit or stand in an upright posture.
- Raise your arms straight up over your head, holding your palms together.
- Bend to your right. Hold for a count of five.
- Bend to your left. Hold for a count of five.

41. Torso Side Bends

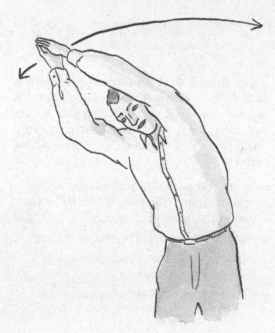

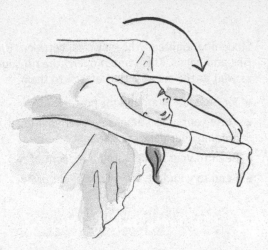

42. Head Over Bed

If you sit at a desk, this exercise is a terrific end-of-the-day antidote for tense muscles. Let gravity assist you in stretching the tissues that tend to get tight as the day progresses. You'll open your chest muscles and breathe better.

- Lie on your back across a bed, stretching your body out. (If this position strains your lower back, bend your knees.)
- Hang your head over the edge of the bed.
- Lift your arms, and extend them over your head next to your ears.
- Hold for a count of ten and exhale.

7

Your Lower Back

"My back is killing me!" is a complaint I hear a lot. That's not surprising, since lower-back pain is incredibly prevalent, especially when people are stressed. A whopping 80 percent of the U.S. population will experience an aching back at some point in their lives. For many of these men and women, pain strikes when they are still in their thirties and forties.

Stress plays a huge role in lower-back pain. Whenever you are frightened or nervous, your body's sympathetic nervous system responds with a "fight or flight" reaction—regardless of whether the threat is real or imagined—with the result that muscles in the lower back tighten, causing painful spasms. As was the case with the mid-back, deep breathing can do a lot to release tension and pain in the lower back (see pages 103–4).

Mechanical strains due to poor posture often team up with stress to cause problems. If you sit with your back rounded, or if you slouch for long periods of time, your spine is going to adapt to those positions and change—and not for the better! Hunching over and slouching compress the muscles, tendons, joints, and ligaments that support the lumbar, or lower, spine. The *lumbar spine* is a support system that extends from the rib cage to the pelvis and includes the muscles of the abdomen and the muscles that attach from the front of the spine and anchor it to the hips. If you persist in hunching over or slouching, eventually your ability to stand or sit upright will be compromised. Just look how hunched over old people tend to become.

Slouching puts more pressure and stress on the disks of the lower spine than any other posture. Over time this can lead to premature degeneration of the disks, a very painful condition. Slouching also causes pain by impinging on the nerves that exit the spinal cord through the lower spine. That's why it's important to keep a normal *lordosis*, which looks like a C-curve-shaped hollow at the lower spine, as much of the time as possible when you are sitting. The negative effects of slouching go beyond the disks and nerves of the lower back, causing misalignments of the bones in that area, too. The bones of the lower back include the five lumbar vertebrae, the five fused segments of the *sacrum* (onto which the pelvis anchors), and the *coccyx*, or tailbone. Sitting correctly helps keep all these bones properly aligned, with each one bearing the full weight of the one above it. (Proper alignment also helps build bone mass because of the weight-bearing of bone on bone.)

Certain physical activities can lead to pain because they make you prone to asymmetries, in which muscles on one side of the spine become short and tight, and those on the other side long and weak. For instance, your tennis or golf swing rotates your spine in one direction over and over again. Even if you just sleep on one side all the time, the muscles on that side of your spine constantly shorten while their counterparts lengthen.

Some low-back discomfort results from injuries to the disks between the five lumbar vertebrae (the vertebrae of the lower back). These disks, which are made up of fibrocartilage, act as large cushions between the vertebrae, absorbing the impact of motion. But if you bend and twist while lifting, you put such intense force on the disks that one or more may be forced to bulge out between the vertebrae above and below. The resulting *disk herniation* can range in severity from bulging to prolapse, and the effects can range from lower-back pain to foot dropping to loss of bladder control, the most serious symptom.

As you get older, the consistency of the nuclei of the disks—the gelatinous material that pushes against the outer cartilage rings—changes, becoming drier and less elastic. The result is that when pressure on the disk causes it to protrude, it does not bounce back as easily as it once did. That's why it takes at least three days for a thirty-to-forty-year-old person to recover from a herniated disk but just twenty-four hours for a twenty-year-old.

Another effect of aging is that the facet surfaces—the two bony surfaces of each vertebra that fit together like Lego pieces—erode from excessive wear and tear, and over time they may fall off track. When that happens, the spinal nerves, which exit the spinal cord through the tripod formed by the two facets and the disk, can be impinged, giving you pain in the lower back or down a leg.

A spine that is strong, aligned, and healthy allows you to flex, extend, and rotate your lower back without "diskomfort." And that's the kind of spine that the Brill exercises will help you create. These movements encourage an adequate flow of blood to the disks, which promotes healing and prevents scar tissue from entrapping the nerves. The nerves get a clear pathway to transmit electrical impulses, allowing the muscles and ligaments to function optimally. This in turn will help ensure that the bones of your spine are in their ideal alignment and the joints in their proper place.

The result will be a stable trunk that supports supple limbs—no matter how stressful your situation. Pain disappears. The Brill exercises give you the ability to treat what can hurt you before pathology sets in. *Instant Relief* proves that you *can* defy the aging process.

Strong Abs Make a Strong Back

One way of strengthening your back is to exercise your abdominal muscles. That doesn't mean performing endless crunches, sit-ups, or curls—these movements create too much pressure on the lower back and cause friction on the vertebrae, making them wear down that much faster. Instead, check out Belly Blasters, Dead Bugs, and the Mermaid—Brill abdominal exercises found in *The Core Program*. They will give you strong abs and protect your back.

43. Standing Backward Bend

This is an incredibly effective move. I've found that 90 percent of people who complain of aching lower backs get relief with this one exercise.

- Stand with your legs a shoulder-width apart.
- Place your hands on your buttocks, with your fingers pointing downward.
- Stretch backward as far as you comfortably can, with your face lifted toward the ceiling.
- Return upright slowly.
- Repeat ten times trying to bend a little further backward with each repetition.

If doing this movement causes any dizziness, don't bend your head back so that it faces the ceiling. Instead, keep your head straight up, with your face forward.

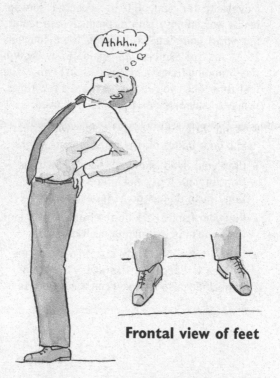

Frontal view of feet

44. Forward Bend

If you are among the 10 percent of people who don't get relief by bending backward, this is the movement for you. But if repeated forward bends worsen your pain or produce pain radiating down your leg, stop doing them immediately and try Exercise 43 again. Even though the Standing Backward Bend didn't work the first time, once you've bent forward a few times, it may finally give you the relief you need.

- Stand with your legs a shoulder-width apart and your hands on the front of your thighs.

- Drop your head. Run your hands down the front of your legs, reaching for the floor. Don't push it; just go as far as you can.

- Run your hands back up the front of your legs until you're in a standing position again.

- Repeat ten times. Try to stretch a little more with each repetition. The goal is to obtain normal range so that you can touch your toes.

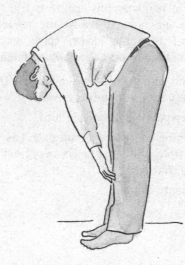

45. Standing Side Glides

If done properly, this maneuver shifts your *pelvis* from side to side but not your *trunk*, thereby isolating the lower segments of the spine—namely the fourth and fifth vertebrae of the lumbar spine and the top of the sacrum. The disks between these particular vertebrae are the most likely to herniate. This maneuver also helps to relieve pressure on the sciatic nerve, which emerges from the lumbar spine and passes through the buttocks and down each leg.

- Stand with your legs a shoulder-width apart with your feet pointing forward.
- Place your hands on your hips.
- Keeping your spine as motionless as possible, shift your pelvis away from the side that hurts.
- Repeat ten times.

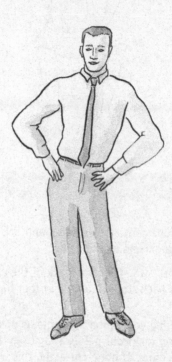

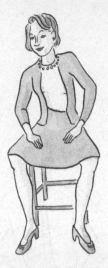

46. Pelvic Shift

This movement also isolates and activates the lower segments of the spine.

- Sit up, away from the back of the chair, with your back straight and your feet flat on the floor.
- Keeping your spine as stable as possible, gently rock your pelvis away from the side that hurts. If done correctly, this will cause your trunk to bend slightly in the opposite direction—in other words, *toward* the side that hurts.
- Repeat ten times.

This movement will ease lower-back pain and tone the abdominal muscles at the same time.

- Sit up straight. Your back can be against the chair. Keep your feet flat on the floor.
- Suck in your belly, pulling your navel toward your spine.
- When you've pulled in your belly as far as you can, hold the position and pulse your belly in quickly for the count of ten. (To maximize the effect, work up to ten repetitions.)

You can also do this exercise standing with your back against a wall. Plant your feet about two and a half feet in front of you and bend your knees as you squat down. Suck in your belly, and continue as above.

47. Transverse Abdominus Back Stabilizer

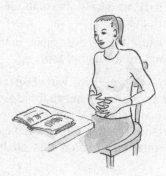

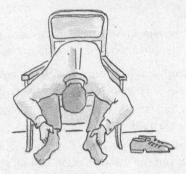

48. Bent-Over Ankle Pull

This movement flexes your spine, which will open up your lumbar spine maximally so that the disks are less likely to be compressed. It will also restore full flexibility to the lumbar spine.

- Sit on the edge of a chair with your knees as far apart as is comfortable, and your feet flat on the floor.
- Reach down between your legs, stretching your back maximally, and grab the outside of each ankle.
- Pull yourself down even more. Hold the position for a count of ten.

Follow this exercise with Exercise 49, the Pelvic Rock. A movement that flexes the spine, like this one, should always be followed by one that extends the spine. That will prevent a disk from herniating, if it has that predisposition.

- Sit up, away from the back of the chair, with your back straight and your feet flat on the floor.
- Slump down, then straighten up again, creating that C-curve hollow in the small of your back that I described on page 112.
- Repeat ten times.

If you feel odd about doing this movement in public, try this variation: slump once, then sit up straight and hold this position for a count of ten. Then relax.

49. Pelvic Rock

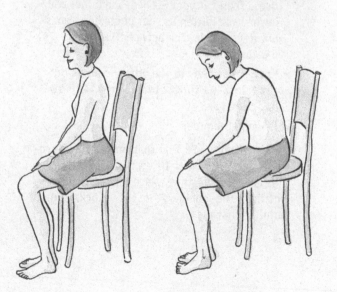

50. Pelvic Clock

If you suffer from lower-back or buttock pain, this exercise will restore normal range of motion in the area where the back meets the pelvis and bring your muscles into balance. If you've been limping or favoring one side, it will help put your back in alignment so that you can walk without pain.

- Lie on your back, and bend your knees. Think of the top of your pubic bone as 6 o'clock and your navel as 12 o'clock and the sides of your pelvis as 3 and 9 o'clock.

- Arch your back—you'll feel your tailbone press into the bed or floor as your navel rises. Then tilt your pelvis—you'll feel your lower back flatten as your pubic bone goes up. Repeat this rock between 12 and 6 o'clock five times.

- Rock your pelvis to the other numbers on the "clock": 1 to 7, 2 to 8, 3 to 9, 4 to 10, and 5 to 11.

- Reverse the order.

Very likely you'll find that one of the movements will be harder to do than the others—the muscles in that place are "stuck." By "hitting" the numbers on the "clock," you'll mobilize that area.

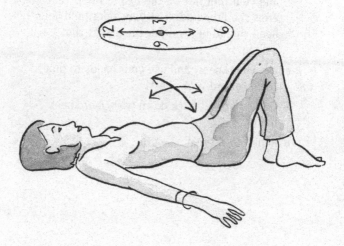

51. Knees to Chest

This movement will open up the facets (the bony contact points in the vertebrae) of the lumbar spine, stretch connective tissues and muscles and aid circulation.

- Lie flat on your back with your knees bent and your feet flat on the bed or floor. Your arms should be down at your sides, and your head should be straight, looking at the ceiling.
- Lift your knees, and use your hands to pull them toward your chest.
- Drop your feet back down with your knees bent.
- Repeat ten times.

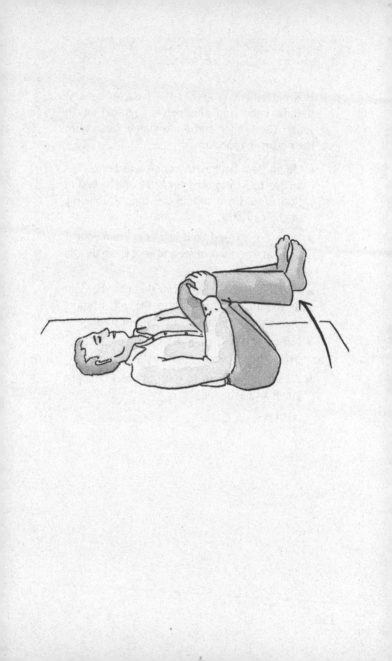

52. Lying Spinal Twist

This movement stretches the muscles between the rib cage and the pelvis, elongating the spine. The longer and more supple your spine, the better it functions.

- Lie on your back with your knees bent, ankles touching, and feet flat on the bed or floor. Your head should be straight, looking at the ceiling.

- Make a T: extend your arms out from your body at shoulder level and rest them on the bed or floor.

- Lift your knees, then drop them to the right as you rotate your head to the left, keeping your shoulders flat on the bed or floor.

- Lift your knees, then drop them to the left as you rotate your head to the right.

- Alternate twisting to the right and left, five times to each side.

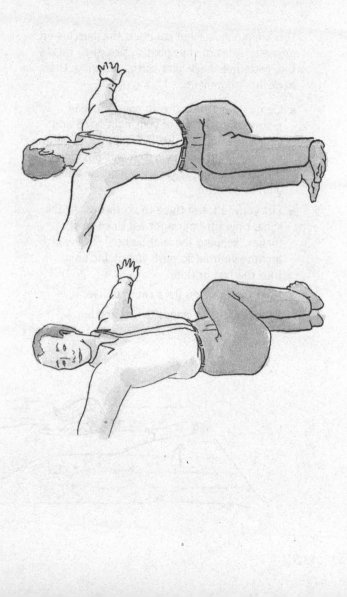

53. Crossed Extension

This simple movement contracts the muscles on opposite sides of the spine so that they rotate the vertebrae back and forth, bringing them back into alignment.

- Lie on your stomach with your forehead resting on the back of your right hand and your left arm extended in front of you, palm down, resting on the bed. If this position is difficult for you, try putting a pillow under your abdomen.

- Lift your left arm three to six inches. At the same time lift your right leg three to six inches, keeping the toes pointed. To avoid arching your back, push your pubic bone into the bed or floor.

- Hold the position for a count of five.

- Repeat with the opposite arm and leg.

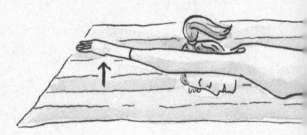

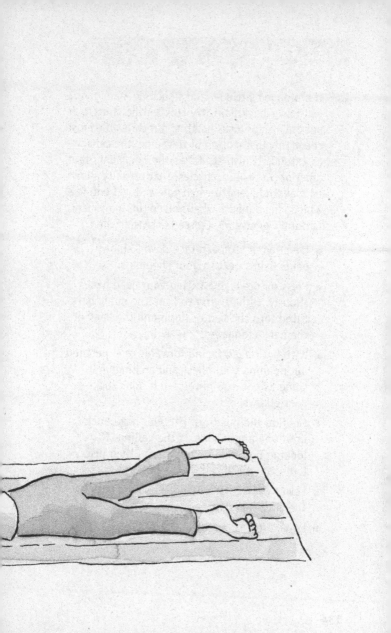

54. Cobra

If prolonged sitting—and slouching—are giving you lower-back pain, try this terrific stretch. It not only keeps disks healthy, it restores the most commonly lost motion of the spine, the capacity to extend. It also stretches the commonly taut anterior (front) hip muscles. That capacity allows normal stride length when you walk. (If you feel a pinch in your back when you do this movement, perform Exercise 53, Crossed Extension, first.)

- Lie on your stomach face down, elbows bent, palms next to your shoulders.

- Press up gradually, tilting your head back slightly, while trying to keep the pubic bone tilted into the bed or floor, and the back of the neck elongated.

- With your head facing forward, keep pushing up, opening your chest and arching your spine as you straighten—but don't lock—your elbows.

- Holding the position, tilt your head back until you are looking at the ceiling. If looking up produces neck pain, then just look straight ahead.

- Lower yourself slowly until you are back at the starting position.

- Repeat ten times

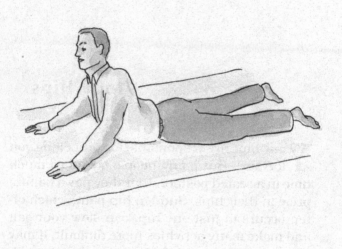

Your Hips

Your hips are responsible for propelling you forward. But many people spend so much time in a seated position that they pay a painful price in their hips. Sudden hip pain, which often occurs in just one hip, can slow your gait and make many activities more difficult. It may also cause you to think that you're getting old, because you no longer have the mobility in your hips that you used to have. This kind of pain is not an inevitable part of the aging process, however. Think about it: if your pain is in only one hip, it doesn't make sense to believe *that* hip is old and the other isn't. Our bodies age symmetrically. The fact that they don't always *work* symmetrically is due to muscle imbalances—the muscle imbalances that occur because of our sedentary lives. Hip pain can also sometimes be traced to asymmetries and imbalances that occur because we favor one hip over the other, as can happen in various sports activities, such as tennis and basketball.

In my physical therapy practice I address hip problems that range from mild to severe; people whose pain halts their running or walking, and post-operative patients who are recovering from fractures (usually women) or total joint replacement due to severe arthritis (usually men). They all get relief from the Brill exercises, which stretch muscles that get tight and strengthen muscles that get weak. The Brill exercises will work for you, too. They will keep your hip joints in proper alignment so that you can move through your day pain-free and with vigor.

Typically, hip joint pain is felt in the groin or in the front or the inside of the thigh. Hip problems, which may also be experienced as back pain and tend to worsen with walking, are usually evident from the way the person walks. First, the knee on the same side as the affected hip stays bent during all phases of gait. (This compensation throws the knee joint off its axis of rotation and can eventually lead to arthritis in the knee. See pages 166–68.) Second, the person will typically step more lightly and briefly on the affected side, in order to shift weight from the hip that hurts. Third, if the hip is stiff due to tight muscles or joint cartilage changes, the torso won't be stable, and the whole trunk of the body will swing forward along with the involved leg.

Although a lot can go wrong with the hip joints, they are actually incredibly strong, stable structures, which are responsible for absorbing at least one and a half times your body weight whenever you walk and three and a half times your body weight when you run. They have a ball-and-socket configuration, with the ball consisting of the head of the *femur*, the longest bone in the body, and the socket formed by the three bones of the pelvis.

Twenty-two muscles surround the hip joint, providing strength and power. These muscles are divided into four anatomical groups that provide for movement in three planes of motion: flexion and extension, abduction and adduction, and internal and external rotation.

The four anatomical hip muscle groups are:

- The anterior, or front, group, which is responsible for flexing the hip
- The inner group, which is responsible for adducting (inwardly rotating) the hip
- The posterior, or back, group, which is responsible for extending the hip
- The outer group, which is responsible for abducting (outwardly rotating) the hip

All four groups work together to stabilize the pelvis as the hip rotates through its very extensive axis of motion. But because our lifestyles are so sedentary, the muscle groups often become imbalanced. Seated postures lead to the shortening of the anterior group, especially the *hip flexor* muscles, the weakening of the posterior group, particularly the *gluteus maximus* muscle and hamstrings, and also the weakening of the outer muscle group, especially the *gluteus medius*. Hip pain results when imbalances—which are inequalities in strength between muscle groups that oppose one another—shift the inherently stable hip joint off its normal axis of rotation.

For example, as the main stabilizing muscle of the pelvis, the gluteus medius needs to be strong in order to counter the very powerful iliotibial band, the muscle that opposes it. The iliotibial band causes an inner rotation of the femur, the bone that extends from the hip to the knee. If the iliotibial band dominates the gluteus medius, it will turn the femur too far inward, throwing both the hip and knee joints off their correct axis of rotation. Shortening of the hip flexors, the muscles that come off the front of the lumbar spine and attach to the hip, also causes problems that result in hip and lower-back pain. Your stride becomes shorter and, over time, the tightness in the hip flexors can contribute to the hunched-over posture seen in elderly people.

Doing a lot of walking optimizes the way nature intended our hips and pelvis to move. But many people must sit for long periods of time and find it difficult to carve out the time for a quick restorative walk. That's why the Brill exercises are so convenient to have at your disposal. For men, who tend to have strong and stable joints, stretching movements will help increase flexibility. For women, who are frequently flexible almost to the extent of instability at their joint surfaces and thus are particularly prone to having joints shifted off the proper axis of rotation, the movements help to build muscle strength. Achieving a balance between suppleness and strength is critical for the hip joint—and every joint. So give yourself a realignment tune-up whenever you're feeling creaky. Even a new car needs one after a certain number of miles.

The exercises in this chapter stretch the muscles around the hip joints. Doing these Brill exercises, you'll knock out pain, move more efficiently, and help your bones and joints absorb the impact of bearing your weight the way they should. I've found that the first one works best for most people who feel pain in the hip while standing or walking. But you may respond better to one of the other exercises. Try them all to see which ones work best for you. And remember, even if the instructions tell you to do the exercise "on the side that hurts," doing it on both sides will mean you get pain relief now *and* pain prevention for the future.

The sciatic nerve runs through the piriformis, the big muscle that extends from the sacral portion of the lower spine to the hip. Runners and cyclists often feel tightness in the piriformis muscle. This rotational maneuver stretches the piriformis and relieves achiness in the buttocks, too.

- With your legs shoulder-width apart, stand a foot or so away from a chair (or other surface you can hold on to), positioning yourself so that the side that hurts is next to the chair.

- Holding on to the chair for balance, bend and raise that knee.

- Using the opposite hand, pull the knee across your body so that the side of the hip gets a good stretch. Keep the standing leg and hip stationary.

- Hold the position for a count of ten.

55. Standing Piriformis Stretch

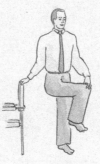

56. Standing Iliotibial Band Stretch

Originating on the side of the pelvis, the *iliotibial band* is a broad muscle with a very long tendon that extends down to the side of the knee. If pain hits you in the hips or the knees, it may be because your iliotibial band, which crosses both those joints, is tight. Pain in the kneecap when you descend or ascend stairs is often the first clue to iliotibial band–related knee trouble.

- If your left knee or hip hurts, place your left hand on the back of a chair.

- Wrap your left foot behind the right foot and keep it flat on the floor.

- Tilt your pelvis to flatten your lower back, and lean into your left hip. You'll feel a stretch down the side of your left leg.

- Hold the position for a count of ten.

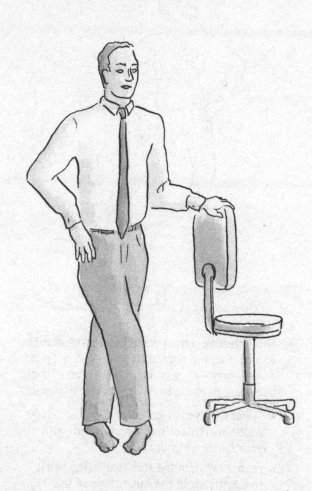

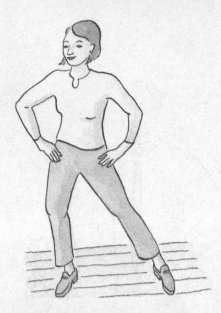

57. Straddle Stretch

This effective action stretches all the muscles around the hip joints. If you hear a "pop," don't worry—it just means that your pubic bones are popping back into proper alignment.

- Stand with your legs wider than shoulder-width apart, feet pointing forward, with your hands on your hips.
- Lean away from the side that hurts; you'll feel a stretch in the inner thigh of that leg.
- Hold the position for a count of ten.

The quadriceps and the hip flexors, the muscle groups in the front of the hips, often get tight from sitting. This movement stretches out those muscles. (If it doesn't work for you, try the sitting version, Exercise 63, Seated Lunge.)

- If it's your left hip that hurts, place your right leg approximately three feet in front of the left, keeping both feet flat on the floor and the toes pointing in the same direction.

- Lunge forward until your right knee is directly over your ankle. Tilt your pelvis up and back. You'll feel a stretch in the front of the thigh of the left leg.

- Hold the position for a count of ten.

58. Lunge and Tilt

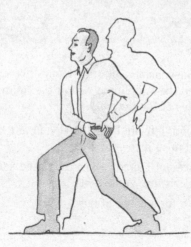

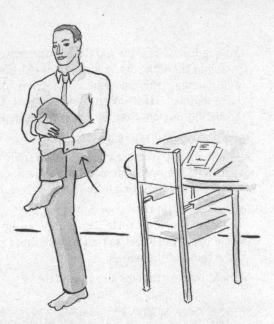

59. Standing One Knee to Chest

This movement will stretch out the cartilage around the hip joint as well as the "glutes," the muscles of the buttocks.

- If your left hip hurts, bend your left knee, and raise it to your chest.
- Place both hands below the raised knee, and press it into your chest.
- Hold for a count of ten.

Hip Help

If hip pain attacks you when you're trapped in a seat—whether at work, in a car, or at a movie—Exercises 60, 61, and 62 will allow you to take action to relieve it right away, without ever leaving your seat.

60. Sitting Tailor

Have you ever seen a tailor sit? Very often tailors rest the ankle of one leg over the opposite knee as they work. Hence the names of the two variations of this pose. (The second one, Reclining Tailor, is Exercise 65.) Both of these movements open the hips and stretch the rotator muscles, giving you increased range of motion in the joint and thereby ensuring adequate blood circulation in that area. As a result, the hip muscles will become supple and strong, better able to generate power and absorb impact.

- Sit up straight, and cross the ankle of the leg that hurts over the opposite knee.
- Place your hands on the top knee, and press down for a count of ten.

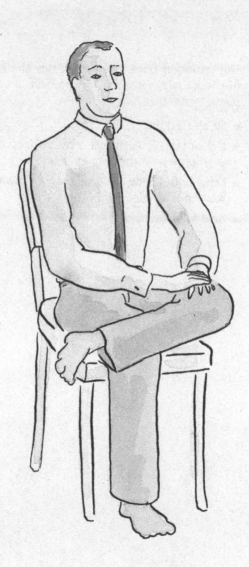

61. Seated Piriformis Stretch

This variation once again elongates the piriformis muscle, releasing the pressure on the sciatic nerve that runs through it.

- Sit up straight.
- If your left hip hurts, place the ankle of your left leg on the right knee.
- Using both hands, pull the left knee toward your right shoulder.
- Hold for a count of ten.

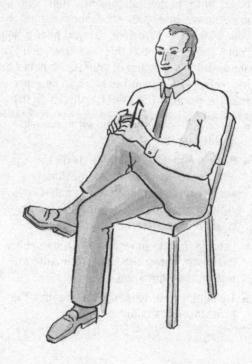

62. Shotgun Technique

In this isometric technique your inner thigh muscles contract maximally to pull your pelvic bones into proper alignment. That will put more power into your stride and ensure that your walking is pain-free. (If you hear a huge "pop" when you do this exercise, don't be alarmed. It's the sound of your pelvic bones being realigned—a sound so much to be expected that the name of the exercise alludes to it.)

- Sit on the edge of a chair with your legs slightly apart.
- Place the palms of your hands on the outsides of your knees, and push out against the resistance of your palms, without allowing any movement, for the count of five.
- Place your left elbow on the inside of your left thigh, above the knee. Your palm will rest on the right knee.
- Try pulling your legs together against the resistance for a count of five.

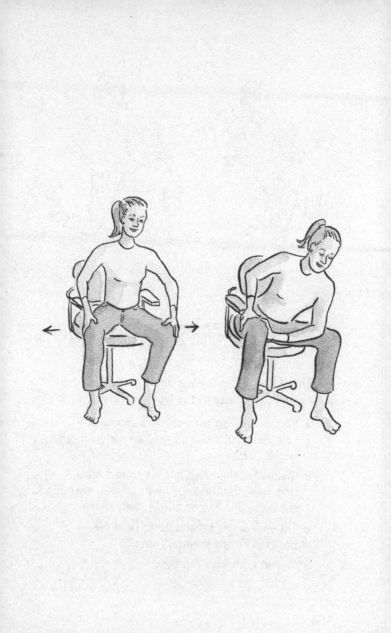

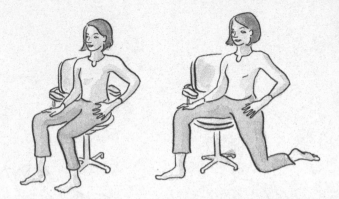

63. Seated Lunge

This movement will ease tightness in the quadriceps, the muscle at the front of the hip.

- Sit sideways on the edge of a chair, with your right buttock on the chair and your left slightly off.
- Gradually lower your left leg toward the floor, keeping the knee bent, until it reaches the floor, and extend the leg behind you.
- Tilt your pelvis up and back. Hold the position for the count of ten.
- Repeat with your right leg.

- Lie on your back with your knees bent and your feet flat on the bed or floor.
- Let your knees fall open, and bring the soles of your feet together. This will give a good stretch to your inner thighs. For a more intense stretch, use your hands to press down gently on your thighs, opening them further.
- Hold the position for a count of ten.

64. Lying Inner Thigh Stretch

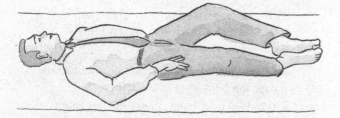

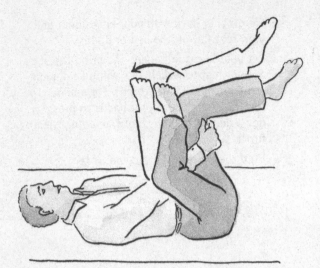

65. Reclining Tailor

With this exercise you can give your hips a much-needed stretch and watch television at the same time (if you like).

- Lie on your back, and cross your right ankle over the bent knee of the left leg.
- Interlace your hands under the left thigh, and pull your knee toward your chest.
- Hold the position for a count of ten.
- Repeat with the left ankle over the right knee.

Here's another way to stretch the cartilage around the hip joint as well as the gluteus muscles.

- Lie on your back. With your right leg extended flat on the bed, bend your left knee, and pull it straight back toward your chest.
- Interlace your hands behind that knee, and gently pull it as close to your chest as you can.
- Hold for a count of ten.
- Repeat with your left leg and right knee.

If you feel a pinch in the groin, this could be a sign that you have degenerative changes in your hip. If the pinch doesn't subside after doing this exercise for two weeks, I suggest you see a physical therapist because you may need hands-on mobilization of the hip joint. The therapist can help you stretch and strengthen the muscles of the hip so that they create optimal alignment of the bones in the hip socket.

66. Lying One Knee to Chest

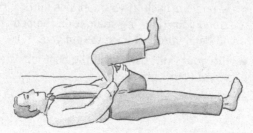

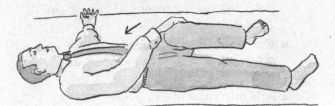

67. Lying Piriformis Stretch

Elongating the big piriformis muscle will relieve discomfort in the hip and buttocks.

- Lie on your back. If your left side hurts, extend your right leg straight on the bed as you bend your left knee toward you.
- With your right hand, pull the bent left knee toward your right shoulder.
- Hold for a count of ten.

This exercise is an excellent way to strengthen the gluteus medius muscle, which attaches from the side of the pelvis into the hip. A toned gluteus medius creates buttocks with good muscle definition, while a weak one will not only allow the buttocks to become flabby but will make you waddle when you walk. Another reason to make sure the gluteus medius is strong is that it will help to prevent osteoarthritis and osteoporosis in the hip.

- Lie on your right side, with your right arm bent so that your hand supports your head.
- Brace your left forearm against your pelvis, supporting it.
- With your left leg on top of your right, bend your knees at a 90-degree angle to your torso.
- Keeping your ankles pressed together, raise and lower your left knee ten times.
- Repeat on the other side.

68. Side Lying Hip Rotations (The Clam)

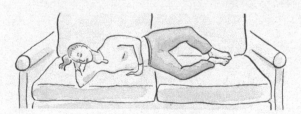

69. One-Sided Cobra

If you feel pain in one buttock, try this movement.

- Lie on a bed, with the painful side of the body right at the edge. Keep your arms bent at your sides and your palms beneath your shoulders.

- Drop the painful leg off the bed, planting the foot firmly on the floor, with the knee slightly bent.

- Lift yourself up onto your elbows, and press up and down, taking care not to lock your elbows, ten times.

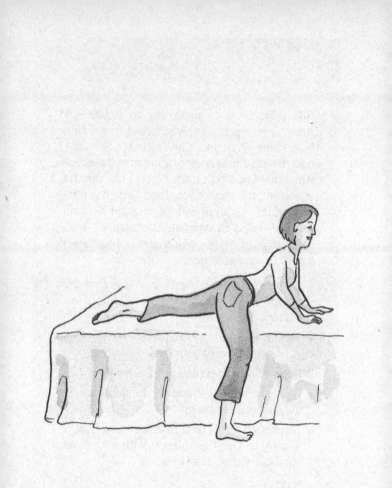

70. Prone Leg Curl (Kick Some Butt)

This exercise is a great way to isolate and stretch the hip flexors, which tend to get tight from hours of sitting, and to stretch the anterior (front) hip muscles while simultaneously strengthening the posterior (back) hip muscles. Stretching the quadriceps, the muscle down the front of the hip joint, will help prevent hip pain. You will feel a tremendous thigh stretch when you do this exercise—you may even be aware of a pull on your abdomen.

- Lie on your stomach with your legs straight behind you. Prop yourself up on both elbows.
- Bend the right knee, and attempt to kick your buttock with your heel.
- Repeat five times, and put the leg down.
- Bend the left knee, and do the same movement, five times.
- Bend both knees, pressing them together, and try to kick the buttocks with both heels, simultaneously, ten times.

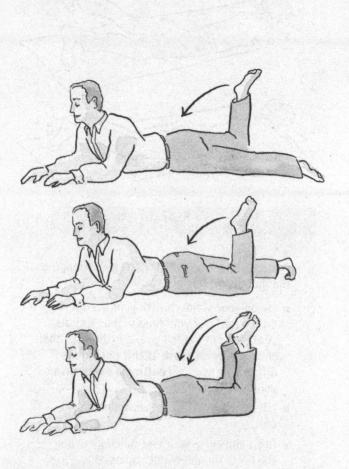

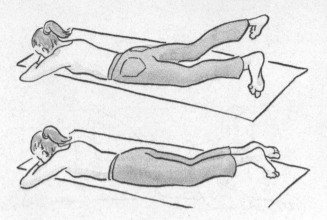

71. Heel Beats

This quick motion will isolate and strengthen the gluteus medius muscle.

- Lie on your stomach with your head resting on the backs of your hands. Your legs are stretched out behind you, a little wider than shoulder-width apart. If this position is difficult for you, try putting a pillow under your abdomen.

- Lift your legs a few inches and flex your feet.

- Open and close your legs quickly, moving the heels shoulder-width apart, then clicking them together.

- Repeat ten times. Keep feet flexed outward through all the repetitions.

Your Knees

Does this sound familiar? You've just finished a long day at the office, racing to meet a deadline and stuck at your desk with almost no time for a break. That night, as you finally descend a flight of stairs to the parking lot, thrilled to be going home at last, you feel a sudden stab of pain around your knee.

Lots of times patients tell me about experiencing sudden knee pain out of the blue. "I did nothing!" they say in bewilderment. But that "nothing" is often at the root of the knee problem. A static posture held for a long time, whether it occurs when you are standing or sitting, results in a muscle imbalance that may be causing your pain. All joints, especially the knee joints, love motion. Even people lucky enough to be born with perfectly healthy knees, which aren't bowed or knock-kneed, are still at risk for sudden knee pain and loss of mobility if their lifestyle consists of sitting for long hours at a desk during the day and spending long hours in front of the TV at night.

Although the most common knee-pain complaint I hear involves walking down stairs, many people also experience knee pain when they sit for long periods of time, or when they get up. Ultimately all these annoyances stem from a muscular imbalance around the knee, which affects how the joint works.

The knee, a weight-bearing joint, is a complicated structure that works like a hinge, with the capacity for a little bit of spin, too. One part of the joint connects the *femur*, or thighbone, which is the longest bone in the body, and the *tibia*, or shinbone. The other part of the joint connects the *patella*, or kneecap, and the femur. The structure of the joint allows for a wide range of knee motion, comprising both flexion and extension as well as the internal and external rotation that allows you to change course in midstride—turning on a planted foot, for instance.

However, when the muscles around the knee are imbalanced, they pull the knee joint away from its axis of rotation. The joint surfaces can't glide and roll around one another as they should. The cartilage that cushions the joint is worn down, with the result that bone rubs against bone, which can be painful. When the cartilage wears away, it no longer produces enough synovial fluid, which is the substance that lubricates the knee joint and allows for friction-free movement. Insufficient synovial fluid will lead to friction that further erodes the cartilage, and all this wear and tear eventually culminates in arthritis.

The knee joint is in the middle of a "seesaw" between all the muscles of the knee. If your knee hasn't sustained an injury but still hurts, the cause may be traced to one or more of the following three types of muscular imbalance, all of which can result from long periods of remaining in static positions. They are:

1. An imbalance between the muscles that control the relationship of the hip to the knee. One muscle, the *tensor fascia lata*, has a very long, powerful tendon, the iliotibial band, which extends from the hip over the knee on the lateral (outer) side. The other muscle, the gluteus medius (located along the upper portion of the buttocks), counteracts the dominant pull of the iliotibial band to assure proper positioning of the femur in relation to the pelvis and tibia. The balanced relationship between these muscles also keeps the pelvis stable over the knee. However, as discussed in the hip chapter, the iliotibial

band sometimes becomes so strong and tight that it dominates knee motion by rotating the thighbone inward. If the gluteus medius is not actively strengthened, you will have difficulty keeping your knee tracking properly during motion, and you will feel pain. (See Exercise 56, Standing Iliotibial Band Stretch.)

2. An imbalance among the three hamstring muscles of the back thigh. The hamstrings extend the hip and flex the knee.

3. An imbalance among the four muscles that make up the quadriceps. The quadriceps extend the knee and flex the hip. These muscles pull on the kneecap to keep it tracking properly in the groove of the femur. Imbalances can also occur between the inner quadriceps muscle and the outer quadriceps muscle. Such imbalances can affect the tracking of the kneecap, with the result that the cartilage behind the kneecap gets pinched. This change in cartilage shows up on X rays and is diagnosed by doctors as *chondromalacia*—another possible source of the pain you feel when you walk up and down steps.

Aside from muscle imbalances, sudden knee pain can also be traced to *hyperextension*. If you tend to keep your knees in a hyperextended position when you are standing, this "locking" may jam your kneecaps into your thighbones, causing the knee to pinch on sensitive cartilage behind the kneecap. Over time, the result may be permanent damage to the cartilage, which leads to arthritis. If you make a point of standing with your "knees at ease," this will help to retrain your muscles to do the work of supporting proper alignment, taking the burden off your knee joints.

Pain is a reminder that you need to adjust your posture. You can get instant relief from sudden knee pain by either contracting or stretching specific muscles in order to restore the normal length and strength of all the muscles around the knee joint. As soon as you feel knee pain, use one or more of the Brill exercises that follow to address it quickly and efficiently. Doing so will keep you from developing a pathology that will limit the mobility of your knee. By making joint motion smooth and pain-free, these exercises also help to enhance the production of synovial fluid, the joint surface lubricant.

Because the knee structure is complex and pain can be the result of many subtle misalignments, I recommend that you try the first exercise in this chapter and progress through all the ones that follow until you get the relief you need. I also recommend doing these exercises on both sides. Your body will thank you.

After you do the exercises in this chapter, I

recommend that you do consistent strengthening exercises for the lower extremities, because strong muscles make for strong joints. Strength training is an important component of keeping the health of your joints optimal. Follow the Ultimate Core in *The Core Program* to keep your lower extremities flexible and strong for a lifetime of mobility.

Ligaments Work Hard, Too

If the quadriceps and hamstrings are in balance and the joint is tracking properly, the ligaments that are crucial for stabilizing the knee—especially the *anterior cruciate ligament* (ACL), the ropelike tissue that crisscrosses behind the knee joint—will be able to do their job. But muscle imbalances, and the resulting misalignments, often put undue stress on the ligaments, especially during sports that involve high impact jumping and cutting movements. Skiers, soccer players, and basketball players often injure their ACL. Women athletes are five times more likely than men athletes to rupture their ACL.

If you experience knee pain while walking down stairs, here is the help you've been waiting for: This movement will strengthen the gluteus medius muscle, which rotates the femur and keeps the kneecap in proper alignment.

- When you feel the knee pain, stop with both feet on one stair.
- Squeeze your buttocks together tightly for a count of ten.
- If the pain persists, keep your buttocks squeezed together as you walk down the rest of the stairs.

72. Squeeze and Step

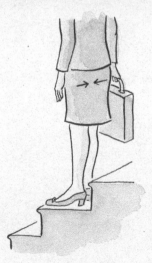

73. Standing Front Thigh Stretch

This exercise helps you to stretch the quadriceps, the muscle that crosses the hip and knee joints. Sitting for long periods of time causes tightness in this muscle.

- Hold on to the back of a chair or place your hand against a wall for balance.
- Bend your left knee back, and reach the foot toward your buttock.
- Take hold of the left foot and slowly pull it toward your buttock, trying to touch your buttock. Hold the position for a count of ten.
- Repeat on the right side.

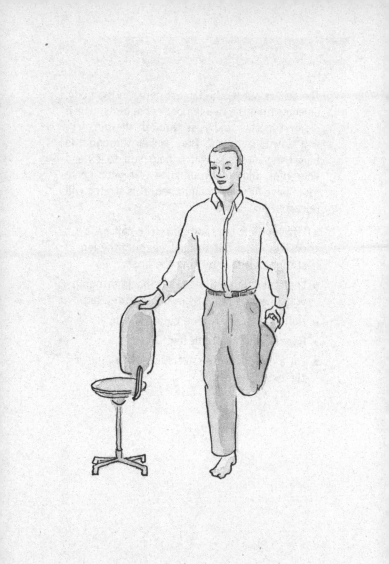

74. Hamstring Stretch

The sciatic nerve, the largest nerve in the body, emerges from the five lumbar nerve roots, which merge together and pass through the buttocks and down each leg. They travel through the hamstring muscles, which help you to extend your hips and flex your knees. If your nerve roots have become compressed, this stretch will release them.

- Lift your left leg, and place the calf on a desk or other flat surface, keeping the leg straight without locking the knee.
- Lean forward with a straight back, bringing your chest as close as possible to the leg.
- Hold the position for a count of ten.
- Repeat with the right leg.
- For a more intense stretch, flex the foot of the extended leg.

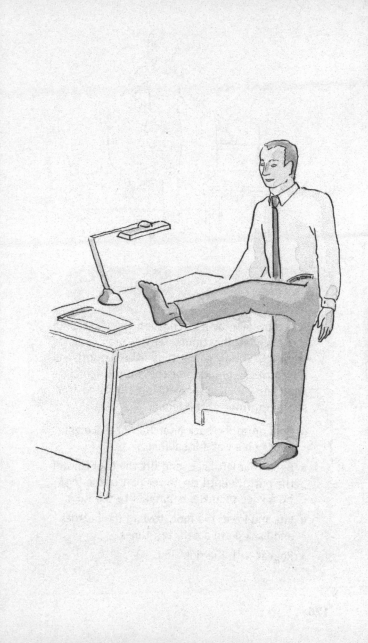

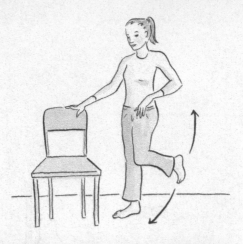

75. Active Hamstring Curls

This movement will strengthen the muscles in the back of the thigh, which provide knee stability. Strong hamstrings also support and reinforce the function of the anterior cruciate ligament (ACL) by preventing the tibia from sliding in front of the femur.

- Hold on to the back of a chair or place your hands on a wall for balance.
- Bend your left knee, and lift the heel toward the buttock until the lower part of the leg, from knee to ankle, is parallel to the floor.
- Lift and lower the foot, toward the buttock and back down again, ten times.
- Repeat with the right leg.

If you do this exercise often enough, you'll be able to squat with your feet flat on the floor, which will give an incredible stretch to the muscles in your hips, knees, and ankles, increasing flexibility in all these areas.

- Hold the inside of a door frame with your arms at shoulder height. Your feet, slightly turned out, should be a bit wider than a shoulder-width apart; your knees should be aligned between the first and second toes.

- Squat down as far as you can, as your hands glide down the door frame. Your heels must remain flat on the floor.

- Hold the position for a count of ten.

76. Deep Squat

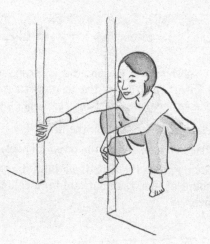

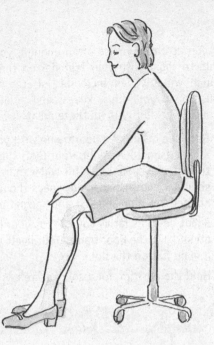

77. Knead and Mobilize

This self-massage loosens the kneecaps around the knee, which helps the tendons to contract and lengthen more effectively for proper tracking.

- Place your feet flat on the floor.
- Place your palms on top of your knees.
- Gently circle the soft tissue inward for a count of five, then outward for a count of five.

This hamstring isometric strengthens the area behind the knee.

- Place your feet flat on the floor.
- Dig your heels down into the floor and lift the toes and top of your feet.
- Hold the position for a count of ten.

78. Dig In Your Heels

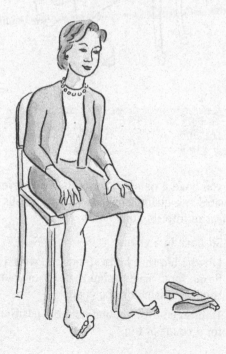

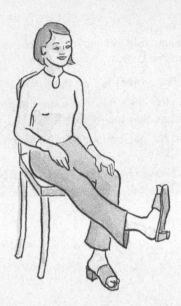

79. Seated Isometric Knee Extension

If you have a painful knee, this nifty move activates the quadriceps muscle, which pulls the kneecap into its proper groove.

- Sit back in a chair.
- Lift the leg that hurts straight up with a flexed foot, making sure the back of your thigh is resting on the chair.
- Tighten your thigh, and hold the position for a count of ten.

This movement, in which gravity will assist you to achieve full knee flexion, will maximize range of motion at your knee joint. And you'll not only be mobilizing a painful knee, but you'll be stretching your hamstring, too.

- Lie flat on your back, and bend the knee that hurts.
- Wrapping your hands behind the thigh of the bent knee, gently pull it toward your chest.
- When the knee is as close to your chest as you can get it, extend (kick) and bend (drop) the leg ten times.

80. Kick and Drop

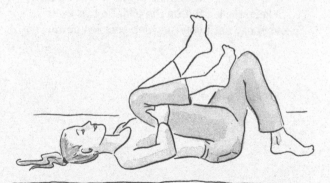

81. Hip Flexor Stretch

If one of your hips hurts, here's an easy way to stretch your hip flexor muscles and iliotibial band. The rectus femoris (one of the four quadriceps) is a hip flexor that crosses the hip and knee joint. Since this joint muscle is important for normal function of both hips and knees, this stretch is great for hip as well as knee problems.

- Lie on your back, on the edge of a bed or even a firm table, and lift your bent knees to your chest.
- Extend the painful leg straight out, keeping it flat on the bed, stretching out the front of the thigh. If the leg drifts outward, bring it back toward the bent leg. Keep your back flat against the bed—don't let it arch.
- Hold the position for a count of ten.

If your hip flexors are tight, it will be hard to keep the leg flat on the bed. Do this exercise every day until you can keep your leg down.

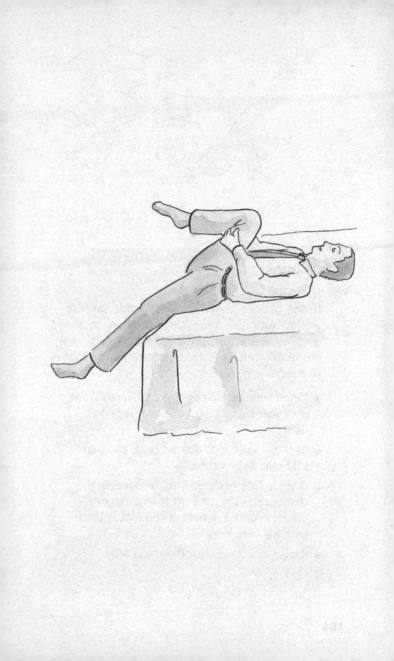

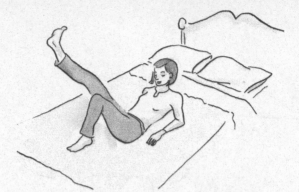

82. Diagonal Straight-Leg Lift

If one of your knees is hurting, this exercise will activate the inner thigh portion of the quadriceps—the vastus medialis oblique (VMO)—which will help pull the kneecap into proper alignment.

- Lie on your back propped up on your elbows with your legs straight out on the bed or floor.
- Bend the knee that doesn't hurt, and place that foot flat on the bed.
- Flex the foot of the painful leg, keeping that leg straight, and lift it in a diagonal direction until the heel of the foot is level with the bent knee.
- Repeat ten times with the thigh fully contracted.

This exercise tones the "glutes" and the hamstrings, two of the muscles that support the knee.

- Lie on your back with your knees bent and your arms by your sides.
- Lift your buttocks off the bed or floor as high as you can, then lower them.
- Repeat ten times.

83. Bridging

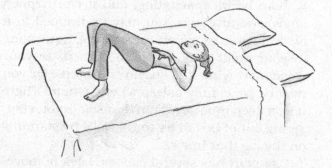

chapter 10

Your Calves

Sudden and severe cramping in your calves can be incapacitating, and it can happen anywhere, anytime. You may be trapped in a chair during an important meeting. Squirming in your chair only seems to exacerbate your discomfort while the spasm continues. Or you may be peacefully asleep when—wham! There it is, a deep muscle cramp that sends you staggering out of bed to try to get relief by standing on the leg that hurts.

Calf pain has several causes. Lack of movement, which inhibits circulation, is high on the list. Dehydration may also be a factor. Your muscles, which are 70 percent water, need a lot of hydration for proper metabolic reactions to occur. But not all liquids are equally good for this purpose. The coffee you drink for the caffeine buzz that keeps you alert and focused, for example, actually has dehydrating effects and may be contributing to your calf cramps. You may not be aware of being dehydrated, but if you suffer from constipation, that's a good indicator that you are.

Poor posture is another possible cause of calf pain, because it compresses certain nerves in the spine as they emerge from the spinal cord. This nerve compression can result in a kind of calf cramp known as *neurogenic intermittent claudication*, characterized by sudden pain when walking; it disappears when you sit down. If this condition persists, it can, over years, lead to serious constraints on your ability to walk, and a permanently bent-over posture. (Do the lower-back movements, Exercises 43 to 54, to keep your spine healthy.)

Muscle imbalances can also cause calf pain. The major calf muscles cross two joints: the knee and the ankle. Four calf muscles (the medial and lateral *gastrocnemius*, the *soleus*, and the *plantaris*) attach to the heel bone via the Achilles tendon.

If you experience calf cramps, take a good look at your legs. Is the skin dry and flaky or discolored? If so, your skin is showing signs of poor blood circulation. Take a look at your toes, too. Do they have hair? They should; hair on the toes is an indicator of good circulation.

Are varicose veins marking blue trails in your legs? They too are symptoms of poor circulation in the lower extremities (although they may also be genetically determined). Tight calves and poor circulation go hand in hand, creating cramps and impeding normal walking.

The Brill exercises in this chapter stretch the protective sheaths that surround the nerves; stretch, strengthen, and balance the calf muscles; and restore normal mobility and strength to the ankle and knee joints. Restoring flexibility and strength to these areas will not only relieve calf pain but will reestablish good circulation and stabilize the ankles, thus preventing ankle sprains in the future.

So the next time a calf cramp hits, you're going to take charge and make it disappear—even if you're sitting in the middle seat on an airplane.

The Core Program

Besides doing the exercises in this chapter, you might want to start on one of the core-strengthening exercise regimens described in my first book, *The Core Program*. Although you may think that the muscles at the core of your body—in the hip, abdomen, and lower-back areas—have no bearing on calf pain, *The Core Program* has helped thousands of people with this problem by restoring flexibility and strength throughout the spine, thus opening up the vertebral segments of the spine from which the nerves that run along the calf emerge.

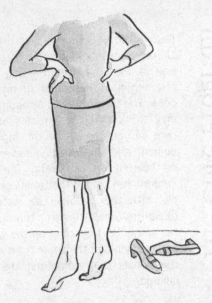

84. Heel Raises, Straight Knees

Have you ever noticed the pronounced calf muscles of dancers? All their exertions strengthen the gastrocnemius muscle, which attaches to the heelbone via the Achilles tendon. The gastrocnemius couples with the hamstring and crosses the back of the knee. Strengthening the gastrocnemius is key for assuring ankle stability. This exercise will help both calf cramps and ankle pain.

- Stand with your feet a shoulder-width apart.
- Raise your heels up and down ten times.

This variation strengthens another calf muscle, the soleus, which is also critical for controlling the ankle. Strong calf muscles help to prevent the outward twisting so commonly responsible for ankle sprains.

- Stand with your feet a shoulder-width apart.
- Bend your knees slightly, and raise your heels. As you raise your heels, imagine that you are squeezing a volleyball between your knees. This will recruit the inner thigh muscles for even greater ankle stability and prevent your ankles from rolling outward.
- Lower and raise your heels ten times.

85. Heel Raises, Bent Knees

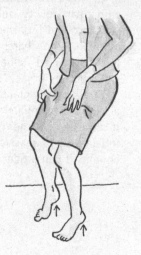

Plantar Fasciitis and Heel Spurs

Plantar fasciitis, a painful condition that can hinder walking and running and doing all kinds of sports, is an inflammation of the thick band of relatively inflexible fibrous material (the *fascia*) that runs along the bottom of the foot, from the heel to the base of the toes. The inflammation is due in part to tightness in the Achilles tendon, which causes you to *overpronate* (flatten) your foot when you walk, so that your feet hit the ground without adequate absorption of impact, as though you were wearing flippers. This strains the fascia and muscles on the bottom of the foot. The result will be heel pain, particularly intense when your foot first hits the floor in the morning. Going barefoot or wearing flat-heeled shoes will only make matters worse.

Stress on the plantar fascia can also result in inflammation where it attaches to the heel. If this inflammatory reaction becomes chronic, it can produce heel spurs.

If you suffer from *plantar fasciitis* or heel spurs, this stretch, which works on the upper part of the Achilles tendon as well as the calf muscles, is for you.

- Extend your arms in front of you at shoulder height, palms flat against a wall.
- If it's your left foot that hurts, position the right leg about one foot in front of the left.
- Tilt your pubic bone and lean toward the wall until you feel a stretch.
- Then hold the position for a count of ten.

86. Wall Stretch (Gastrocnemius)

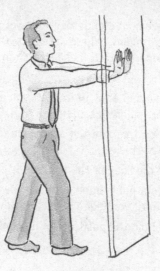

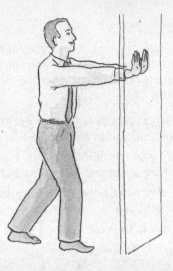

87. Wall Stretch (Soleus)

This movement elongates the lower part of the Achilles tendon, where it meets the heel. If done properly, you'll feel a stretch in your lower left calf.

- Extend your arms in front of you at shoulder height, palms flat against a wall.
- Position the right leg about one foot in front of the left.
- Bend the knee of the left leg.
- Tilt your pubic bone and lean toward the wall until you feel a stretch in your left calf.
- Then hold the position for a count of ten.

Economy-Class Syndrome

If you find yourself sitting in one position for a long period of time—and who doesn't?—your blood circulation is going to be compromised. In extreme cases deep vein thrombosis, better known as "economy-class syndrome," occurs. To prevent that from happening, do the next three movements once an hour when you fly, as well as any time your calves start to cramp. (To give yourself extra "plane" protection, do Exercise 78, Dig In Your Heels, every hour, too.)

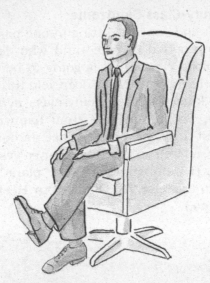

88. Ankle Pump

In this exercise, a great one for preventing or relieving calf cramps, the point-and-flex motion promotes optimum circulation in all the muscles around the calves.

- Sit up straight with your feet flat on the floor.
- Raise your left leg, and extend it to a 45-degree angle.
- Point and flex your foot ten times. Lower the leg.
- Repeat with the right leg.

This movement not only eliminates cramps in calves; it works on toe cramps as well.

- Place your feet flat on the floor.
- Raise your left leg, and extend it to a 45-degree angle.
- Flex your foot until you feel a stretch in your calf.
- Lift your leg up as high as you can while remaining comfortable. Hold the position for a count of ten.
- Repeat with the right leg.

89. Seated Calf Stretch

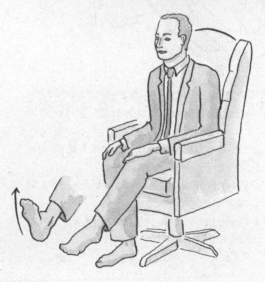

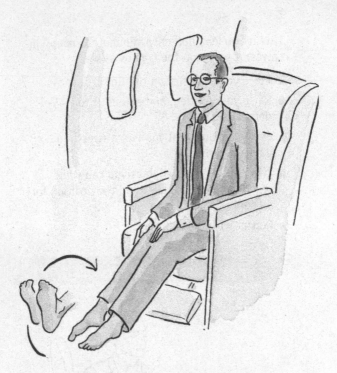

90. Two Ankle Circles

- Sit up straight with your feet flat on the floor.
- Raise both legs, and extend them to a 45-degree angle.
- Circle both ankles to the right five times, then to the left five times.

If calf cramping—better known as charley horse—disturbs your sleep, try doing this exercise when it happens—or better yet, before you close your eyes. Often cramping is due to nerves or blood vessels being entrapped in the calf muscle. Spinal stenosis—the degenerative changes that narrow the spaces through which nerves exit the spinal cord—is another possible cause of pressure on the nerves. Either way this stretch will help.

- Lie on your back with your legs extended on the bed.
- Lift the leg with the cramp straight up to a 90-degree angle, and hold it with both hands behind your knee.
- "Draw" capital letters, from A to J, in the air with the big toe.

91. Foot Writing A to J

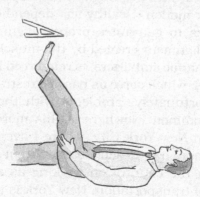

11

Your Feet

Your feet get you where you want to go, so you want to be sure to keep them in optimum working condition: flexible and well-balanced, with a spring to their step and power to their motion. Healthy feet depend on strong muscles to guarantee proper alignment. The good alignment created by the muscles, which are dynamic stabilizers, is reinforced by the ligaments, which serve as passive restraints.

Unfortunately, problems with the feet are very common. Nowhere is this more obvious than in New York City, where I live and work and where people depend more than anywhere else in the country on walking as a primary form of transportation. New York is also home to the fastest walkers in the country. (New York average 3.6 miles an hour, while the rest of the country averages 2.5 miles an hour.) Speed, I'm glad to say, does not cause foot problems—as long as the muscles of your feet are balanced and the bones are in alignment. But often they aren't. I know this because so many patients complain of foot pain.

When everything works right, the twenty-six bones, 107 ligaments, and nineteen muscles in each foot permit optimal movement. Here's an easy way to understand how your feet work. There's a forefoot (the toes), a midfoot (the bones in the middle), and a hindfoot (the heel and the attachment to the ankle). The heel strikes the ground and provides a stable landing, the midfoot absorbs impact, and the toes extend to allow forward propulsion.

Often the muscles become imbalanced, however: some muscles weaken while others become short and tight. Those mechanical stresses put a strain on tendons, ligaments, and joints. Nerve compression follows, as does impeded blood circulation. Add these problems to the daily strains that the feet endure, and it's no surprise that so many of us suffer with sore feet.

Women in particular are prone to certain kinds of problems because of the shoes they like to wear. If you are a woman who wears either backless shoes or styles with heels higher than two inches, consider this: using your toes to grip the inside of the shoes so that they won't fall off causes a strain in your foot muscles. Your normal gait is altered, and all of a sudden your feet hurt. You are also setting yourself up for unattractive and painful foot deformities like bunions, hammertoes, calluses, and corns, as well as plantar fasciitis, heel spurs, and neuromas (nerve irritations that feel like a pebble in a shoe). To compensate, you will take shorter strides, leading to a progressive loss of mobility beginning in the foot and working its way up the leg, hindering the normal motion of the hip.

I do realize that wearing sexy, stylish footwear is sometimes in order. After wearing those fabulous shoes, however, be sure to do these Brill exercises to restore balance to, and relieve stress on, your muscles and joints.

The Brill foot exercises not only relieve sudden foot pain, they can restore optimal function. By stretching what tends to tighten and by strengthening what tends to weaken, they balance the muscles, decompress the nerves, restore mobility, and aid circulation. They will also help to prevent or correct any malformations that may occur. (I got rid of postpartum flat feet and bunions by doing Brill exercises. For antibunion therapy go to Exercise 97, All Toes Up [Active], and Exercise 92, Foot Dome.)

The stretching and strengthening exercises in this chapter will also help to prevent arthritis, which develops when muscle imbalances shift bones out of their proper alignment, causing excessive wear along joint surfaces and ultimately destroying the cartilage between the bones.

If unexpected foot pain slows you down and makes you miserable, these Brill exercises will make you feel better fast. They'll also go a long way toward assuring lifelong foot function—especially if you do them on both sides, not just the side that hurts.

Good Circulation

The Brill exercises in this chapter, which are all done in a sitting position, will promote enhanced blood circulation, lymphatic drainage, and venous blood return. Venous return is particularly important, because it's a long way from the feet to the heart, and your bloodstream must fight gravity the whole way.

If your feet swell, it's because all the fluids that have accumulated in your feet aren't flowing the way they should. These easy movements will bring you relief from swelling and pain. They will also mobilize the foot bones, allowing your joints to move normally. And of course, they will stretch and strengthen muscles. In addition to doing these exercises, make sure you are drinking enough water to assist kidney filtrations (kidney dysfunctions ofen lead to swollen ankles).

You'll see that some of the Brill exercises are

"passive," while one is "active." Passive means that your hands do the work. *Active* means that the muscles of your feet do the work themselves.

Before you do these movements, please take off your shoes.

Give Your Feet a Break

You can help protect your feet by wearing shoes that fit properly. Think of your foot as a triangle formed by the first and fifth toes and the heel. Your shoes should distribute your weight evenly among these three areas. In order to give your feet adequate power for their push-off and good shock-absorption capacity for their landing, your shoes should have adequate space inside to allow them to go through their full range of motion, flexing and extending from heel to ball to toes, and pronating and supinating from side to side as need be.

The toe box should be long enough to allow a space as wide as a thumbnail between the tip of your longest toe and the tip of the shoe, and the shoe should have good arch support. The backs of the shoes should be firm, and the heels, for both men and women, should measure between one and two inches high. Remember to alternate your footwear daily, which will shift any pressure to different muscles, allow for recovery, and prevent cumulative strains to the feet.

92. Foot Dome

Building this "dome" will strengthen the muscles of the transverse arch, which will help the feet absorb impact. You'll also be protecting the fat pads on the bottom of your toes, which cushion your footfall. When those pads are worn down, walking can become painful.

- Stand in your bare feet.
- Take a half step forward with your right foot. Your weight should be mostly on the left foot.
- With your right heel firmly planted on the floor and your toes as straight as possible, raise the top of the right foot so that it looks like a dome.
- Hold the position for a count of ten.
- Repeat with your left foot.

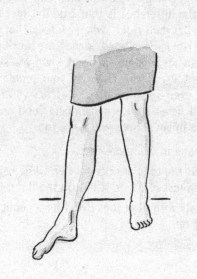

93. Toe-Lift Arch Builder

Many people think they have flat feet. However, true flat feet are a congenital abnormality and are, in fact, quite rare. What most people think of as flat feet are actually feet that have under-developed muscles of the arch. One way you can tell the difference is that true flat feet are not just flat but rigid, whereas feet that simply have underdeveloped arches are flexible, and the arches become apparent when you stand on your toes. If the latter is your problem, this Brill exercise will build the arches you thought you'd never have. (Remember: Good arch supports in your shoes will help, too.)

- Stand in your bare feet.
- Lift the toes of both feet up while keeping the rest of the foot flat on the floor.
- Walk with your toes lifted for a count of ten.

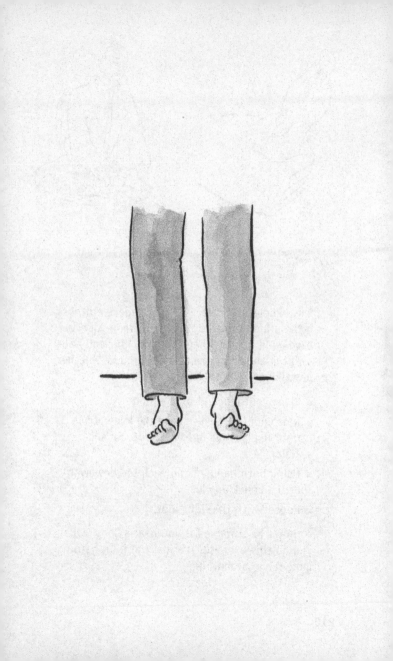

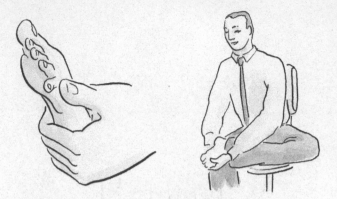

94. Single Toe Curl (Passive)

This simple maneuver will help relieve stiffness by assuring normal foot flexion. When your feet have good flexion, they can more efficiently absorb the impact of meeting the ground, whether in walking, running, or jumping.

- Place your feet flat on the floor.
- Rest your left ankle above the knee of the right leg, just as in Exercise 60, Sitting Tailor.
- Using both hands, bend each toe downward at the knuckle twice.
- Repeat with the right foot.

Don't be surprised if you hear a "pop" when you do this exercise. It's just the joint gaining more range of motion.

This stretch puts joints into their maximal range of motion, restores normal muscle length, and helps prevent arthritis.

- Place your feet flat on the floor.
- Rest your left ankle above the knee of the right leg.
- Grasp the toes of the left foot with your right hand and bend them forward from the base.
- Hold for a count of ten.
- Repeat with the right foot.

95. All Toes Curl (Passive)

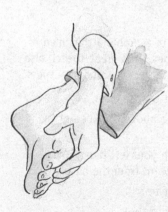 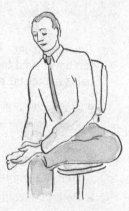

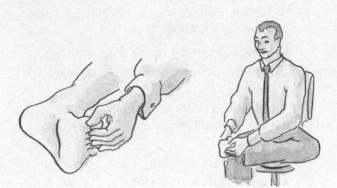

96. All Toes Up (Passive)

This movement targets a problem that men often have: rigid big toes. This great stretch also helps to prevent plantar fasciitis and heel spurs.

- Place your feet flat on the floor.
- Rest your left ankle above the knee of the right leg.
- Grasp the toes with your left hand, and stretch them backward from the base.
- Hold for a count of ten.
- Repeat with the right foot.

This exercise will give you stronger muscles to support the longitudinal arch along your instep, which will help relieve foot pain, especially pain related to bunions.

- Place your feet flat on the floor.
- Lift and splay your toes. Make sure that the bottom of your foot, from the ball to the heels, remains flat on the floor.
- Hold the position for a count of five, and relax.
- Repeat for another count of five.

97. All Toes Up (Active)

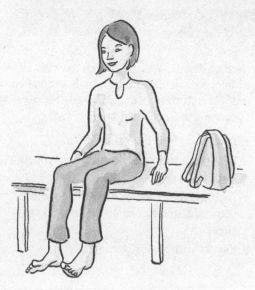

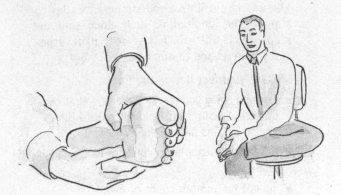

98. Self-Massage

Here's a terrific way to stretch muscles as well as improve circulation, especially venous blood that is returning to the heart for oxygen. Lymphatic drainage will benefit, too.

- Place your feet flat on the floor.
- Rest the left ankle above the knee of the right leg.
- Position your thumbs at the midpoint of your sole, and stroke up and inward ten times.
- Repeat with your right foot.

This lift strengthens the posterior tibialis muscles, the midstance supporters of the feet, and can help relieve foot pain.

- Lie on the side of the foot that hurts, propped up on your elbow with your hand supporting your head.
- Extend the bottom leg and point the foot slightly.
- Bend the top leg, placing the foot in front of your body.
- Moving from the ankle, lift the slightly pointed foot of the bottom leg up and down, with emphasis on the upward motion, ten times.

99. Foot Inverter

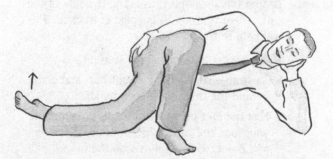

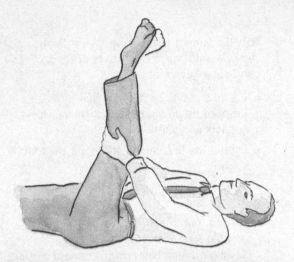

100. Sural Nerve Glide

If you still feel pain from a twisted ankle that has healed, try this exercise. The cause of your discomfort is the sural nerve, which originates behind the knee and runs along the side of the calf, where it tends to become entrapped. This will help to free it.

- Lie flat on your back, legs straight.
- Raise the painful leg straight out, and grab behind the thigh with both hands.
- Flex the foot of the elevated leg, then point your foot and turn it inward. Repeat the flex and point, with emphasis on the inward motion, ten times.

Acknowledgments

S pecial thanks to my devoted husband, Gary, and my two precious daughters, Madison and Maggie, who sacrificed time and attention to let me give you *Instant Relief* and who have always been the most important part of my own health, happiness, and success.

John J. and Christy K. Mack have mentored me in every way and have done more for my soul than I could ever do for their bodies.

I have enormous gratitude to all the patients of Brill Physical Therapy who trust in our care for their physical therapy needs, and who have played the crucial role in my attempts to discover the solutions for optimal recovery and to help people defy the degenerative processes associated with aging.

Certain people must be recognized for their wonderful contributions to me professionally and personally—Mitch Merin, Bob and Karen Scott, Philip Purcell, Ralph Pellechio, Tom Kearns, Kevin Murphy, Dick Fisher, Jeanne Donovan, Lewis Bernard, Brad Evans, José Rivera, David Haynes, Enes Dedovic, Jane Carlin, Paula DeMaggio, Tanya Grubich, Kathy Courtenay, Beatrice Jaye, Lauren Hutton, Lois Feldman, Pattie Sellers, Ann Morfogen, Matthew Sharp, Raymond Granger, Michael Nice, Mike Krzyzewski, Ed Skloot, Madeline Purnell, Philip Tanen, Katie Sosnowski, Patrick Whalen, Vicki Rosen, Judith and John Angelo, Aaron Fuchs, Rustam Dastor, Beverly Taylor, Frank Greenberg, Julie Harris, Jean Galmot, Lisa Einbinder, Svetlana Gutevich, Rick Woolworth, Betty Lok, Larry Mitchell, Janet Nelson, Valerie Malkin, Cheri Baum, Maria Kennedy, James Furey, Michael McGuinness, Stanley Tulin, Nancy Saper, Mady Goldstein, Peter Straus, Kenwyn Dapo, Julie Tupler, Dora Newman, Jackie Castro-Cooper, and Catherine Crier.

I am honored to work with many of the best doctors in the world. I appreciate all your support and trust in Brill Physical Therapy. My gratitude is to Doctors Charles Goodwin, Henry Lodge, Dana Mannor, John Postley, David Case, Jean Case, Henry Birnbaum, Tracey Gaudet, Orrin Sherman, Lewis Maharam, Gerald Varlotta, Paul Greenberg,

Louis Bigliani, David Altchek, Jo Hannafin, Mark Sultan, Frank Petito, and Christiane Northrup.

Herb and Nancy Katz, my literary agents and angels, made magic selling and shaping a vision for health, and have blessed me to the moon and back. Susan Suffes, my writer, gave it all and then some, to clarify medical jargon into reader accessibility, and I thank you for the long hours of dedication you graciously shared.

Many thanks to all those at Bantam who contributed to this project. Beth Rashbaum, my editor extraordinaire, brilliantly dove into every detail until I couldn't imagine loving the book any more than I do—thank you for your beaming enthusiasm. Glen Edelstein and Amanda Kavanagh, I commend you for a fabulous layout and design. Thank you, Meredith Hamilton, for all the charm that your winsome illustrations bring to this book; each speaks a thousand words. Irwyn Applebaum, Bantam's publisher, and Nita Taublib, deputy publisher, are committed to producing an incredible product that readers will adore, and I am grateful.

I thank my treasured friends Tamar Amitay, Maria and Peter Hoelderlin, Fern and Neil Zee, Stephanie Bologa, Melanie Fink, Christine Aragon, Elaine Stillerman, Robert Morton, Gina Rosselli, Christine Bergmann, Christopher Rotondo, Carol and Paul Miller, Paula Pryer, Joanna Andreou, Donna and Brian Baron, Bill and Marianne Jones, Peter Ward, Bonnie Wiseman, Kenneth Wright, Helen and Arthur Gorecki, Jannette Bolger, Ronald and Andrea Ponchak, and Roz Barrow Callahan for all their love and laughter, which have enhanced my life so much.

My devoted staff make work a joy—Jennifer Neisler, Yasminda Hammond, Raymond Masselli, Heather Case, Michael Ingino, Vivian Andujar, and Nolly Tobierre.

About the Authors

PEGGY WACHTERHAUSER BRILL, P.T., is a board-certified clinical specialist in orthopedic physical therapy. Her private practice, Brill Physical Therapy, has three offices, two in midtown Manhattan and one downtown. Her expertise is sought after by the Duke University men's basketball team, top executives all over the world, and leading physicians at the Hospital for Special Surgery and several other major medical centers. The author of *The Core Program: 15 Minutes a Day That Can Change Your Life,* Peggy lives in New York City with her husband and two daughters. Visit her website at *www.brillpt.com.*

SUSAN SUFFES is a writer and editor who lives in New York City.